Manual of Coagulation Disorders

D0863173

Manual of Coagulation Disorders

Michael H. Kroll, MD

Associate Professor of Medicine and
  Molecular Physiology & Biophysics
Baylor College of Medicine
Veterans Affairs Medical Center
Houston, Texas

**Blackwell
Science**

©2001 by Michael H. Kroll

Blackwell Science, Inc.

Editorial Offices: Commerce Place, 350 Main Street, Malden, Massachusetts 02148, USA
Osney Mead, Oxford OX2 0EL, England
25 John Street, London WC1N 2BS, England
23 Ainslie Place, Edinburgh EH3 6AJ, Scotland
54 University Street, Carlton, Victoria 3053, Australia

Other Editorial Offices:

Blackwell Wissenschafts-Verlag GmbH, Kurfürstendamm 57, 10707 Berlin,
Germany
Blackwell Science KK, MG Kodenmacho Building, 7-10
Kodenmacho Nihombashi, Chuo-ku, Tokyo 104, Japan
Iowa State University Press, A Blackwell Science Company, 2121
S. State Avenue, Ames, Iowa 50014-8300, USA

Distributors: *The Americas* Blackwell Publishing
c/o AIDC
P.O. Box 20
50 Winter Sport Lane
Williston, VT 05495-0020
(Telephone orders: 800-216-2522;
fax orders: 802-864-7626)

Australia Blackwell Science Pty, Ltd.
54 University Street
Carlton, Victoria 3053
(Telephone orders: 03-9347-0300;
fax orders: 03-9349-3016)

Outside The Americas and Australia
Blackwell Science, Ltd.
c/o Marston Book Services, Ltd.
P.O. Box 269
Abingdon
Oxon OX14 4YN
England
(Telephone orders: 44-01235-465500;
fax orders: 44-01235-465555)

Acquisitions: Laura DeYoung
Development: Angela Gagliano
Production: Irene Herlihy
Manufacturing: Lisa Flanagan
Marketing Manager: Toni Fournier
Cover design by Meral Dabcovich, VisPer
Typeset by Best-set Typesetter Ltd., Hong Kong
Printed and bound by Sheridan Books, Inc.

Printed in the United States of America
03 04 5 4 3 2

Library of Congress Cataloging-in-Publication Data

Kroll, Michael H.
  Manual of coagulation disorders / by Michael H. Kroll.
    p. ; cm.
  ISBN 0-86542-446-2
  1. Blood coagulation disorders—Handbooks, manuals, etc. I. Kroll, Michael H. II. Title.
  [DNLM: 1. Blood Coagulation Disorders. 2. Anticoagulants—therapeutic use. 3. Embolism. 4. Fibrinolytic Agents—therapeutic use. 5. Platelet Aggregation Inhibitors—therapeutic use. 6. Thrombosis. WH 322 K93m 2001]
  RC647.C55 K76 2001
  616.1′57—dc21

                                                                                    2001025053

This work is dedicated to my teachers, my students, and my wife and children—
Penny and Samantha, Jeffrey, and Caleb.

Around 610 AD a solitary man wandering the world in search of a vocation
experienced an epiphany. This event is referred to as "The Night of Destiny."
Somewhere in the rock-strewn desert of what is now western Saudi Arabia a
voice called to him, summoning him to recite. The man, Muhammad, replied
"What shall I recite?" The voice said:

> In the name of thy Lord who created,
> Created man of a blood clot.
> And thy Lord is the most bountiful,
> Who taught by the pen,
> Taught man what he knew not.
> (Qur'an 96:1–5)

Table of Contents

Notice: The indications and dosages of all drugs in this book have been recommended in the medical literature and conform to the practices of the general community. The medications described and treatment prescriptions suggested do not necessarily have specific approval by the Food and Drug Administration for use in the diseases and dosages for which they are recommended. The package insert for each drug should be consulted for use and dosage as approved by the FDA. Because standards for usage change, it is advisable to keep abreast of revised recommendations, particularly those concerning new drugs.

Preface

The evaluation of patients with hemorrhage or thrombosis often yields a precise diagnosis leading to a specific and effective therapeutic intervention. This is because the history, physical examination, and laboratory testing flow logically from an understanding of basic mechanisms of coagulation. There are few classes of diseases, in fact, that provide a better example of how basic scientific discoveries are translated into routine clinical practice; or of how clinical observations can be investigated in research laboratories to yield new diagnostic and therapeutic approaches. The interdigitation of clinical and laboratory medicine in the field of hemostasis and thrombosis has a long tradition dating back to 1854 and Rudolf Virchow's description of a "triad" of *blood, blood vessel, and blood flow* as elements in the pathogenesis of thrombosis. More recent developments such as Born's invention of the platelet aggregometer in 1962, Macfarlane's "cascade" and Davies and Ratnoff's "waterfall" hypotheses of coagulation, both published in 1964, were rapidly incorporated into the mindset of a diverse group of investigators to yield much of the foundation for current medical practice. Since then, the field has moved very far, very fast; in most cases its progress has followed pathways presaged by Virchow over a century ago. In the past three decades extensive information has been catalogued about blood, vascular, and rheological factors that regulate physiological hemostasis or pathological hemorrhage and thrombosis. This information derives from the thoughtful and creative efforts of clinicians, clinician-scientists, and scientists. Their efforts have led to all of the concepts presented in this book, and make hopeful all endeavors to elucidate those phenomena currently not understood.

Acknowledgments

I thank Drs. Penny Jaffe and Glen Levine for critically reading several chapters, June Osterholm and Fay Houston for assistance with manuscript preparation, and Lynn McLemore, R.Ph., for help with drug information. I also thank Christopher Davis, Angela Gagliano, and Irene Herlihy from Blackwell for their assistance during the different phases of publication.

M. H. K.

1

Mechanisms of Coagulation

Coagulation pathways are important, and it is therefore reasonable to expect students of coagulation disorders to have thorough knowledge of the reactions leading to fibrin and platelet deposition. Outside of the context of clinical experiences, however, the importance of coagulation reactions is never immediately apparent. Thus, it is risky to place the reaction pathways at the beginning of a syllabus or book devoted to coagulation disorders—the only applause I have ever received in a lecture on the subject is when I've announced that I am wrapping up! Therefore, the following text should be used mainly as reference material. Knowledge of coagulation pathways is certainly the foundation for understanding clinical disorders of hemostasis and thrombosis, but it is a foundation that is best constructed carefully and gradually by a process that fits the give and take between clinical phenomena and human biology, which is so nicely developed in this field of medicine.

Coagulation Schemes

There are two major defense mechanisms against bleeding: fibrin generation and platelet aggregation. These two responses to blood vessel injury operate in concert, although fibrin generation may be relatively more important for hemostasis in veins and venules, and platelet aggregation may be relatively more important for hemostasis in arteries, arterioles, and capillaries. Coagulation can be physiological (hemostasis) or pathological (thrombosis). In both cases, coagulation is initiated when the endothelium of a blood vessel is damaged, resulting in the exposure of blood to subendothelial constituents. The subendothelium contains smooth muscle cells and fibroblasts that express tissue factor, an integral cell membrane protein that, under blood flow conditions present in veins and venules, initiates coagulation reactions culminating in fibrin production (Fig. 1.1). It also contains extracellular matrix proteins (e.g., collagen) that, under blood flow conditions that develop in arteries and the arterial microcirculation, bind directly to platelets and bind to plasma von Willebrand factor (vWF), which then attaches to platelets streaming rapidly past the area of vascular endothelial injury. Collagen and vWF binding to circulating platelets

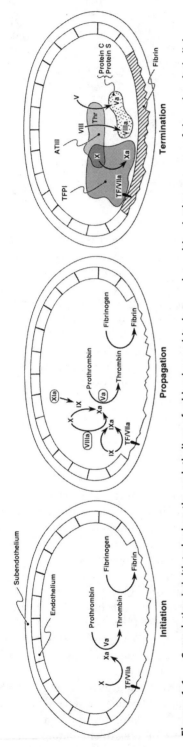

Figure 1.1.   Coagulation is initiated when the endothelium of a blood vessel is damaged, resulting in the exposure of the subendothelial constituents, such as smooth muscle cells and fibroblasts. Tissue factor (TF) is an integral membrane protein constitutively expressed on subendothelial cells, and when it is exposed to blood, it complexes with circulating factor VII (FVII). The TF/FVII (or more likely TF complexed with activated FVII [FVIIa]) is the critical *initiating* reaction that ultimately results in fibrin generation. For this to occur, the TF/FVIIa complex cleaves the proenzyme FX to FXa, which complexes with the cofactor FVa to form the "prothrombinase" complex, which converts prothrombin to thrombin. Thrombin then cleaves soluble fibrinogen, releasing fibrinopeptides A and B, and generating insoluble fibrin. The *propagation* phase develops 1) from TF/FVII–catalyzed FIX activation and 2) from small amounts of thrombin generated by the initiation phase. The TF/FVIIa complex proteolytically cleaves the proenzyme FIX to FIXa, which in the presence of the cofactor FVIIIa causes FX activation. FXa then activates the prothrombinase complex as described above. In addition, not shown is that thrombin cleaves the proenzyme FXI to FXIa, which cleaves FIX to FIXa, leading to FX activation and enhanced production of the prothrombinase complex resulting in fibrin formation. Thrombin-catalyzed proteolysis is also responsible for generating the activated cofactors FVIIIa and FVa. The circled factors are those activated by thrombin. The *termination* phase develops rapidly to limit the extent of fibrin formation, and is mediated by a series of natural anticoagulant proteins. Tissue factor pathway inhibitor (TFPI) complexes with FVIIa and FXa, terminating the initiation reaction. Antithrombin III (ATIII) binds to and inactivates thrombin and FXa. Activated protein C, in conjunction with its cofactor protein S, inactivates the cofactors FVa and FVIIIa. The coagulation response is therefore shut off and fibrin is deposited only where it is needed to plug the injured vessel.

results in platelet adhesion, a process that initiates a series of cellular responses culminating in platelet thrombus formation (Fig. 1.2).

The current model of blood coagulation differs from the original "waterfall" or "cascade" schema, in which an "intrinsic pathway" begins with contact activation of factor XII (FXII), leading to FIX activation followed by FIX and FX activation; and an alternate "extrinsic pathway" initiated by tissue factor (TF) and FVII activation, also leading to FX activation (Fig. 1.3). The primary ambiguity of the old model was the importance of FXII, because clinical bleeding among persons affected by severe hereditary FXII deficiency is entirely absent (see Chapter 17). In contrast, it is known that some patients with FXI deficiency have a severe bleeding disorder when provoked, indicating FXI's importance in normal hemostasis. The current model reconciles these clinical observations

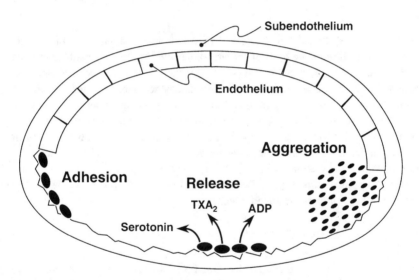

Figure 1.2. Platelets may be the primary defense against hemorrhage in the arterial circulation, where elevated blood flow limits fibrin deposition (leading to a "white thrombus"). Platelets adhere to exposed subendothelium (*adhesion*), secrete proaggregatory and vasoactive substances such as serotonin, thromboxane A_2 (TXA$_2$) and ADP (*release*), and aggregate to form a plug at the site of vascular endothelial injury (*aggregation*). They also contribute to fibrin ("red thrombus") generation in the venous circulation. The coagulation reactions that result in fibrin production are enhanced by cell surfaces, and platelets are an important site of assembly of the coagulation apparatus, particularly the "tenase" (FXIa, FVIIIa, and calcium) and "prothrombinase" (FXa, FVa, and calcium) complexes. The importance of these (and other) phospholipid surfaces is dramatized by experiments showing that the kinetics of these reactions in the absence of membrane phospholipids are so slow that they are physiologically meaningless. Activated platelets may be particularly good sites of coagulation reactions, as they express receptors for certain coagulation proteins (FV, FVIII) and, under some conditions, release microparticles that carry the assembled prothrombinase complex.

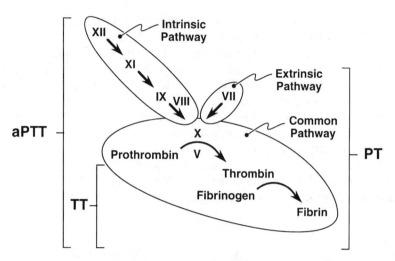

Figure 1.3.   The "cascade" or "waterfall" model of blood coagulation is of more than historic interest. It forms the basis of current laboratory measures of coagulation function. The activated partial thromboplastin time (aPTT) is the time it takes blood to clot after clay is added to recalcified EDTA-anticoagulated blood. Clay activates FXII, and thus the aPTT measures the activity of proteins of the intrinsic pathway and everything downstream, including the common pathway. The prothrombin time (PT), from which the INR (international normalized ratio) is derived, is the time it takes for thromboplastin to clot blood. Thromboplastin is a brain homogenate rich in tissue factor, and PT is thus a measure of the activity of the extrinsic pathway, as well as the common pathway and the subsequent propagation phase (see Fig. 1.1). The thrombin time (TT) measures the time for blood to clot after thrombin is added directly.

with laboratory data, and concludes that FXII is irrelevant to FXI activation in vivo. Rather, FXI is activated by small amounts of thrombin generated during the TF/FVII–mediated initiation phase (see Fig. 1.1). Thus activated, FXI amplifies the coagulation machinery through the intrinsic pathway.

Endothelium and the Vessel Wall

The coagulation reactions associated with hemostasis and thrombosis take place within the framework of Virchow's triad, and thus one must consider the influence of the blood vessel and blood flow on mechanisms of thrombin generation and platelet activation shown in Figures 1.1 and 1.2. The blood vessel, by the constitutive and stimulated production of specific molecules, has the capacity to effect either antithrombotic or prothrombotic responses. As described previously, the smooth muscle cells and fibroblasts of the subendothelium constitutively produce TF. In addition, the vascular endothelium can be induced to synthesize TF by inflammatory cytokines, endotoxin, and certain growth

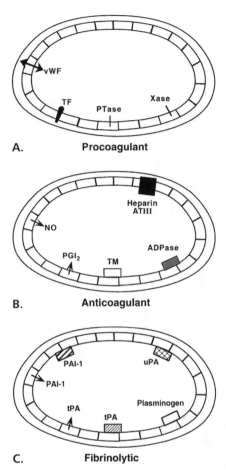

Figure 1.4. The intact vascular endothelium has procoagulant, anticoagulant, and fibrinolytic properties. (**A**) *Procoagulant.* It can rapidly secrete stored von Willebrand factor (vWF), and its plasma membrane provides a scaffolding upon which the prothrombinase and tenase complexes are assembled; within a few hours after cytokines or growth factor stimulation, it expresses active tissue factor. (**B**) *Anticoagulant.* Its antiplatelet properties include the constitutive production of nitric oxide (NO) and ADPase activity, and the induced synthesis of prostacyclin; its anticoagulant function include constitutive and stimulated thrombomodulin production (which is required for the generation of activated protein C), as well as localized heparin/antithrombin III complexes that inhibit factors X and thrombin. (**C**) *Fibrinolytic.* The vessel wall secretes tPA and plasminogen activator inhibitor-1 (PAI-1), and endothelium binds these molecules as well as plasminogen and urokinase-type plasminogen activator (uPA).

factors. The vascular endothelium is a source of vWF, which is released constitutively, and can also be secreted in large amounts when these cells are stimulated by substances such as thrombin, histamine, and DDAVP. The vascular endothelium is also the site of assembly of the "tenase" and "prothrombinase" complexes, thereby enhancing the in vivo rate of catalysis of FX and prothrombin to levels that are physiologically meaningful (Fig. 1.4A).

Opposing the procoagulant function of the disturbed vessel wall is a number of anticoagulant properties (see Fig. 1.4B). Endothelial cells (ECs) secrete nitric oxide (NO) and prostacyclin (PGI$_2$), both of which inhibit platelet aggregation and relax vascular smooth muscle. They also express an ecto-ADPase (adenosine diphosphatase) that breaks down extracellular adenosine diphosphate (ADP), an important stimulator of platelet aggregation. ECs constitutively express thrombomodulin, which binds thrombin and enhances thrombin-mediated cleavage of protein C to activated protein C (see Fig. 1.1). The vessel wall subendothelium contains heparin-like molecules (heparan proteoglycans) that bind to antithrombin III (ATIII) and thereby enhance its inhibitory activity towards thrombin, FIX, FX, and FXI.

The vascular wall participates in fibrinolysis (see Fig. 1.4C). The endothelium is the site of synthesis of tissue plasminogen activator (tPA) and plasminogen activator inhibitor-1 (PAI-1), and it binds tPA, urokinase-type plasminogen activator, and plasminogen. The subendothelial extracellular matrix binds plasminogen and accumulates PAI-1 secreted abluminally by the overlying endothelium. The functional consequences of these in vitro observations to in vivo coagulation remain uncertain, but it is reasonable to speculate that the regional balance between profibrinolytic and antifibrinolytic factors localizes fibrinolytic activity to areas of intact endothelium, thereby limiting fibrin deposition to sites of vascular injury.

Rheology

It is useful to consider the nature of blood flow within our vascular circuit. Blood flow depends on many factors, including blood pressure, vessel compliance, vessel diameter, vessel branching, and blood viscosity. In general, there is comparable blood flow (measured in volume/unit time) in the arterial and venous circuits. There are not, however, comparable flow velocities (distance/unit time) in arteries and veins, and the differences in arterial versus venous flow velocities account for the differences in the composition of venous versus arterial thrombi: venous thrombi are composed predominantly of fibrin and red cells ("red thrombus") and arterial thrombi are composed primarily of platelets ("white thrombus"). Why is this?

Arteries have flow velocities that are relatively high, resulting in elevated shear stress on the vascular wall. Shear stress is the friction (force per unit surface area [dyn/cm^2]) between laminae, and blood flow can be considered an infinite number of infinitesimal laminae, each suffering a frictional interaction with its neighbor. Within a roughly tubular vessel, blood flow generates a parabolic flow velocity profile: at the center of the tube, the flow velocity is maximal and shear stress is minimal, whereas at the blood–tube interface (the vessel wall), the flow velocity is minimal and shear stress is maximal (Fig. 1.5). The wall shear stress/viscosity = wall shear rate (cm/sec per cm or sec^{-1}), and different blood vessels demonstrate different shear stresses or shear rates (Table 1.1).

The shear stress generated by blood flow, because it is a frictional force between blood and the blood vessel, affects the coagulation reactions taking place at sites of vascular injury. In the venous circulation, where shear stresses are low, the activation of the coagulation factors can develop without being "washed away" by the force of the flowing blood on the vessel wall. In the arterial circulation, the higher shear stresses associated with increased flow tend to dilute out certain procoagulant molecules, such as fibrinogen and perhaps prothrombin and thrombin, thereby preventing the formation of insoluble fibrin. To circumvent this interesting dilemma, a system has evolved in which a "super-

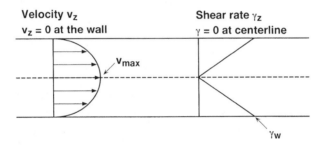

Figure 1.5. Blood flow in a tubular chamber generates a parabolic flow velocity profile. This results in maximal velocity and minimal shear at the center of the blood flow stream, and minimal velocity and maximal shear at the vessel wall. It is the difference in velocity between laminae of flowing blood that generates shearing forces. (Reprinted with permission from Kroll MH, Hellums JD, McIntire LV, et al. Platelets and shear stress. Blood 1996;88:1525–1541. © American Society of Hematology, 1996.)

Table 1.1 Typical ranges of wall shear rates and wall shear stresses

BLOOD VESSEL	WALL SHEAR RATE (/s)	WALL SHEAR STRESS (dyn/cm²)
Large arteries	300–800	11.4–30.4
Arterioles	500–1600	19.0–60.8
Veins	20–200	0.76–7.60
Stenotic vessels	800–10,000	30.4–380.0

Reproduced with permission from Loscalzo J, Schafer AI, eds. Thrombosis and hemorrhage. 2nd ed. Philadelphia: Lippincott Williams & Wilkins, 1998:370. Copyright © 1998, Lippincott Williams & Wilkins Co.

glue-like" bridging ligand (vWF) supports platelet adhesion and aggregation on subendothelial structures exposed in injured vessels, even in the face of extremely elevated wall shear stresses. The arterial thrombus represents a dynamic rheological process, however: as luminal diameter decreases, so does blood flow and flow velocity, such that fibrin generation ultimately develops. The activation of the soluble coagulation systems is a secondary but significant event in pathological arterial thrombosis.

2

The Biological Basis for Routine Coagulation Testing

Many of the biological principles that govern the coagulation system have been translated into clinically relevant laboratory systems useful for patient care. These tests are employed routinely (i.e., PT, aPTT, and platelet count), or are used to evaluate select patients with a bleeding diathesis (i.e., the von Willebrand disease screen) or a "thrombophilic" (hypercoagulable) state (i.e., the activated protein C resistance workup). The usefulness of testing within the context of specific differential diagnoses will be examined in some detail throughout the remainder of this book. What follows is a simplified explanation of tests listed in Tables 2.1 and 2.2, which are available to diagnose and manage patients with hemorrhagic or thrombotic disorders. A more detailed review is offered elsewhere (1).

The Bleeding Patient

First Tier Testing

The prothrombin time (PT) and activated partial thromboplastin time (aPTT) reflect reactions schematized in Figure 1.3. These tests represent the first line of screening for patients suspected of a hemorrhagic disorder due to an abnormality in fibrin generation. Both tests are automated, but consist basically of the recalcification (adding calcium) of citrate-anticoagulated blood ("blue top tube") followed by the addition of a reagent that initiates the coagulation reaction. For the PT, the reagent is tissue thromboplastin enriched in *tissue factor*, which complexes with factor VII and triggers the extrinsic pathway of factor X activation. For the aPTT, the reagent is clay, which activates factor XII and initiates the intrinsic pathway of coagulation.

Heterogeneity in the potency of commercially available thromboplastins leads to a lack of uniformity in PT measurements in a single laboratory over time, and in laboratories from different institutions. This has resulted in

Table 2.1   Laboratory investigation of the bleeding patient

	FIRST TIER	SECOND TIER	THIRD TIER	FOURTH TIER
Coagulation factor disorder	PT	Mixing studies	vWF antigen	Lysis by urea
	aPTT	D-dimer (or FDPs)	Ristocetin cofactor	vWF multimers
	Thrombin time	Reptilase time	Factor levels	α_2-antiplasmin level
Platelet disorder	Platelet count	Bleeding time	[^{14}C] Serotonin release	
		Platelet aggregation	Electron microscopy	

Table 2.2   Laboratory investigation of the thrombophilic patient

	FIRST TIER	SECOND TIER	THIRD TIER
Coagulation factor disorder	APC dysfunction	Protein C level	Heparin cofactor II
	Factor V Leiden mutation	Protein S level	Plasminogen
	Prothrombin G20210A	Antithrombin III level	
	Dilute RVVT		
	Antiphospholipid antibody titer		
Platelet disorder	Heparin-associated antibody		
Vascular disorder	Plasma homocysteine level		
Mixed disorder	DIC screen: platelet count,		
	PT, aPTT, D-dimers, blood		
	smear, TTP: CBC, blood		
	smear, PT, aPTT, LDH		

Abbreviations: DIC = disseminated intravascular coagulation; RVVT = Russell's viper venom time.

the institution of the *international normalized ratio* (INR). The INR = $(PT_{PATIENT}/PT_{CONTROL})^{ISI}$, where the ISI is the *international sensitivity index* of thromboplastin used in the coagulation laboratory. This is discussed further in Chapter 5.

The platelet count is routinely provided with most automated complete blood counts (CBCs). It is important to determine that the platelet count is not artifactually low due to platelet clumping that occurs when EDTA (and to a lesser extent citrate) anticoagulated blood specimens sit around before use. This *pseudothrombocytopenia* is confirmed by observing platelet clumps on the stained blood smear, and by platelet count normalization when it is measured in blood anticoagulated with heparin. The basis for this phenomenon appears to be spontaneous activation developing when platelets are kept suspended in calcium-free solutions (see Chapter 14).

Second Tier Testing

The second tier tests used to investigate bleeding include *mixing studies*. These are used to distinguish a coagulation factor deficiency from a coagulation factor inhibitor. Because 50% of any coagulation protein is sufficient to support a normal PT and aPTT, an abnormal PT and/or aPTT will correct when equal volumes of a patient's and a normal donor's plasma are mixed *when there is a factor deficiency.* On the other hand, when there is an inhibitor (usually an antibody against a coagulation factor; see Chapter 18), the coagulation studies will not correct. This is because *the inhibitor inhibits the coagulation factor in the mixture, whether it is derived from the patient's plasma or the normal control plasma.*

The most common inhibitors discovered during the workup of an abnormal aPTT are *lupus anticoagulants.* These are a heterogeneous group of antibodies that inhibit phospholipid-dependent in vitro coagulation reactions (e.g., the *tenase* or *prothrombinase* reactions), thereby leading to an elevated aPTT (and sometimes an elevated PT), but they are usually *not* associated with bleeding. The most common type of lupus anticoagulant is an antibody that recognizes the complex formed by a plasma protein termed β_2-*glycoprotein I*, with a cell membrane anionic phospholipid such as cardiolipin. Not all of these antibodies are lupus anticoagulants, however, because not all cause abnormalities of coagulation tests; in other words, all lupus anticoagulants are antiphospholipid antibodies, but not all antiphospholipid antibodies are lupus anticoagulants. In certain settings, lupus anticoagulants and isolated antiphospholipid antibodies are associated with thrombosis (see Chapter 9). A lupus anticoagulant should be sought in asymptomatic or thrombophilic patients whose elevated aPTT does not correct with mixing. A variety of tests are available to establish the presence of an antiphospholipid antibody that interferes with in vitro coagulation. Perhaps the best functional test, in terms of standardization and availability, is the *dilute Russell's viper venom time* (DRVVT), in which a low concentration of snake venom is added to recalcified blood to initiate coagulation. This dilute venom weakly activates the "tenase complex" (FIX, FVIII, FX, calcium, and phospholipid; see Fig. 1.1), and a low titer (or weakly avid) antiphospholipid antibody will prolong the DRVVT. Antiphospholipid antibodies that do not affect in vitro coagulation tests (and thus are *not* lupus anticoagulants) can be associated with recurrent thrombosis (see Chapter 9); these are measured directly using a solid-phase immunoassay, such as an anticardiolipin ELISA (enzyme-linked immunoabsorbent assay).

D-dimers come from plasmin-digested cross-linked fibrin. *Fibrin split (or degradation) products* come from plasmin digestion of polymerized fibrin. Both are greatly elevated in disseminated intravascular coagulation (DIC), and can be found at moderately high levels among patients with large thromboses or with liver disease (the liver is the site of clearance of D-dimers and other fibrin degradation products). They are measured by simple immunoassay using an antibody specific for an epitope found only on plasmin-digested cross-linked fibrin.

The *thrombin time* is generated when thrombin is added to recalcified blood. Therefore, it simply measures the conversion of soluble fibrinogen to insoluble fibrin clot. Most things that prolong the thrombin time also prolong the PT and aPTT (as the conversion of fibrinogen to fibrin is the final phase of the common pathway measured by both PT and aPTT). Dysfibrinogenemia, which is the synthesis of a functionally defective fibrinogen molecule (as in liver disease) typically causes an elevated thrombin time. Heparin, fibrin degradation products, and paraproteins also elevate the thrombin time. A mixture of snake venoms that directly cleaves fibrinogen to fibrin can be added to plasma to cause clot formation. This reaction is not inhibitable by heparin, and a normal *reptilase time*, in the setting of an elevated thrombin time, indicates an overt or occult heparin effect.

The *bleeding time* is a measure of the platelet-vessel wall interactions schematized in Figure 1.2. It is very useful when it is done properly in the appropriate setting. For example, it can be very useful for evaluating bleeding patients whose first tier tests have been normal. IT SHOULD NEVER BE USED FOR ROUTINE PREOPERATIVE SCREENING IN ANYONE WHO IS WITHOUT A PERSONAL OR FAMILY HISTORY OF BLEEDING. In this setting it is without any prognostic significance. Recognizing that the bleeding time serves no purpose as a screening test avoids undue anxiety or treatment delays (2). The bleeding time is particularly useful for guiding diagnostic studies directed at qualitative platelet disorders (Chapter 15) and von Willebrand disease (Chapter 16).

Third and Fourth Tier Testing

Third and fourth tier tests are directed at pinpointing a specific cause of a bleeding disorder. Thus, they are best used to examine abnormalities discovered on first and second tier testing. Figure 2.1 provides an algorithm for investigating an elevated aPTT, as an example of how testing is done sequentially, with one result leading down a certain testing pathway.

Coagulation factor levels are usually assayed by *functional tests*. The patient's plasma is mixed with plasma from an individual with a known factor deficiency, and the correction of the elevated study (PT, aPTT, or thrombin time) is absent if the patient is also deficient in that coagulation factor. The relative quantity of deficient factor in a patient's plasma can be determined by examining the effect of dilution of that plasma mixed 1:1 with deficient plasma (thus, if a 1:2 dilution corrects, but a 1:10 doesn't correct, your patient's plasma contains between 5% and 25% of normal factor activity). Coagulation factor protein mass can also be measured using an immunological assay, such as an ELISA. A normal quantity of factor associated with decreased activity defines a *qualitative* problem with the factor, such as a mutation affecting the enzymatic activity of a coagulation factor (e.g., a variety of point mutations affecting factor IX) or abnormal post-transcriptional biosynthesis affecting the properties of a substrate (e.g., fibrinogen in liver disease).

A special functional test for von Willebrand factor (vWF) is the *ristocetin cofactor assay*. Ristocetin is a large molecule originally developed as a macrolide antibiotic (like erythromycin). It induces vWF to bind to platelets and cause aggregation. The ristocetin cofactor assay tests the ability of vWF from

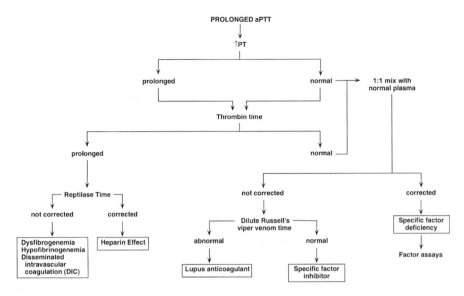

Figure 2.1. A simplified algorithm for evaluating a patient with an elevated aPTT.

a patient's plasma to support ristocetin-induced aggregation. Store-bought platelets (lyophilized or formalin-fixed) are mixed with a patient's platelet-poor plasma (PPP; derived by centrifugation of platelet-rich plasma) in an aggregometer to which ristocetin is added. If there are sufficient quantities of structurally normal vWF, the mixture will aggregate.

vWF quantity can be measured by immunoassays employing specific antibodies. The multimeric composition of plasma vWF is measured by agarose gel electrophoresis. More details concerning the use of these tests in diagnosing and classifying von Willebrand disease are provided in Chapter 16.

Platelet aggregation studies are routinely available in clinical coagulation laboratories using instruments that measure light transmission. As platelets aggregate, light transmission through the turbid suspension of platelets (in plasma) increases. Usually a series of platelet activating substances are tested (e.g., ADP, epinephrine, collagen, and ristocetin), and the pattern of aggregation responses provides an indication of pathogenesis and diagnosis (see Chapter 15 for additional details).

Other tests are routinely available to investigate uncommon bleeding problems that may be associated with completely normal first and second tier studies. These include *clot lysis in urea*, which measures the stability of the fibrin clot. Fibrin clot stability is affected by factor XIII deficiency, which causes poor covalent cross-linking of single-strand fibrin polymers. An α_2-*antiplasmin deficiency* leads to insufficient inactivation of plasmin and overactive fibrinolysis. Both factor XIII and α_2-antiplasmin deficiencies can lead to clinical bleeding with completely normal first and second tier diagnostic testing.

The Patient with Thrombophilia

Thrombophilia refers to the presence of a hypercoagulable state. This will be discussed in greater detail in Chapter 10. Thrombophilia is an increased tendency to thrombosis due to an ongoing thrombogenic stimulus or a defect of the natural anticoagulant or fibrinolytic machinery, which leads to a tip in the balance of the procoagulant and anticoagulant factors operating within Virchow's triad. There are both genetic and acquired causes of thrombophilia. Genetic causes typically lead to familial syndromes of recurrent thrombosis and/or recurrent thromboses that first present in young adulthood or childhood (e.g., activated protein C resistance from factor V Leiden). Acquired thrombophilias usually present later in life (e.g., antiphospholipid antibody syndrome; see Chapter 9), or occur within a specific clinical setting (e.g., heparin-associated thrombocytopenia with thrombosis, lupus anticoagulants in association with SLE or recurrent spontaneous abortion, and myeloproliferative disorders associated with hepatic vein thrombosis—the Budd-Chiari syndrome).

The pathophysiologic features that distinguish venous thrombosis from arterial thrombosis serve as a reasonable conceptual framework in which to describe the biological basis of laboratory testing for patients with recurrent thrombosis: venous thrombosis is usually due to deficient anticoagulant activity, whereas arterial thrombosis is usually due to a platelet or vascular disorder. The pathogenesis of some clinical conditions is multifactorial, so thromboses are expected to involve both venous and arterial circuits. One example of this is thrombosis associated with lupus anticoagulants. Furthermore, there can sometimes be a mysterious overlap in the vascular distribution of thromboses in clinical syndromes, apparently due to a disturbance in the activity of a protein that functions primarily as a natural anticoagulant. For example, some patients with a deficiency of protein S have arterial thrombosis. A hallmark of many of the inherited thrombophilias is the presence of thrombosis in unusual places, such as the mesenteric, hepatic, portal, and cerebral venous circuits.

The simplest approach to patients suspected of having hereditary thrombophilia is to "play the odds" of diagnostic probabilities when *establishing a diagnosis will impact on your treatment program* (see Chapter 10). The most common diagnosis is activated protein C (APC) deficiency from factor V Leiden, which is diagnosed in 20% to 50% of patients with a history of recurrent venous thrombosis. Hyperhomocystinemia may be the next most common cause of recurrent venous thrombosis (in about 13% of patients), as well as the most common cause of recurrent early onset arterial thrombosis (before 45 years of age, as occurred in 19% of patients in one study [3]). Next in line is prothrombin G20210A (about 6% of patients) followed by protein C deficiency (about 3% of patients). Other thrombophilias leading to venous thrombosis are protein S deficiency (~1%), antithrombin III deficiency (~1%), plasminogen deficiency (<1%), heparin cofactor II deficiency (<1%), and congenital dysfibrinogenemia (leading to a fibrin clot not susceptible to lysis by plasmin). Acquired conditions associated with thrombosis include antiphospholipid antibodies (identified as the cause in about 10% of patients with venous thrombosis). Antiphospholipid antibodies also lead to arterial thrombosis, although these are about half as common as venous thrombosis; interestingly, individual patients tend to get either recurrent venous or arterial thrombosis, but not both.

APC deficiency is associated with venous thromboembolism, and case control studies suggest that it is not associated with arterial thrombosis, particularly myocardial infarction or stroke. In about 80% of cases, APC deficiency is caused by a conserved point mutation in one or both alleles of the factor V gene, leading to an amino acid substitution (glutamine for arginine at position 506 of the mature factor V protein) that renders it resistant to cleavage by protein C. The mutant factor V retains its full coagulant function. The heterozygous state is extremely prevalent in the U.S. population: 3% to 5% of all persons carry the mutant allele. This is a risk factor for venous thrombosis, and women taking oral contraceptives who are carriers of the allele have a greatly increased risk for developing venous thrombosis. The reason why APC resistance leads to venous thrombosis is because activated protein C is incapable of shutting off the essential cofactor factor V, which maintains the activity of the prothrombinase complex (see Fig. 1.1).

APC deficiency is diagnosed by a functional test that measures the increase in the aPTT when APC is added to the reaction mixture (Fig. 2.2). The time to clot is measured over a range of doses of APC, and an *APC ratio* is generated (aPTT with APC/aPTT without APC). The mutation is measured by several

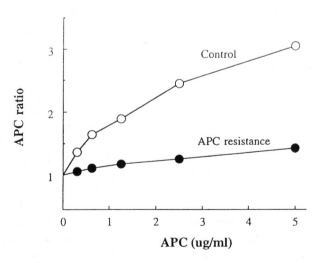

Figure 2.2.   Activated protein C (APC) resistance is evaluated by measuring the aPTT in the presence and absence of a series of doses of APC. The APC ratio is the aPTT in the presence of APC divided by the aPTT in the absence of APC. Note that the APC-resistant person has a blunted dose-response. (Reprinted by permission from Dahlback B. Inherited thrombophilia: resistance to activated protein C as a pathogenic factor of venous thromboembolism. Blood 1995;85:607–614.)

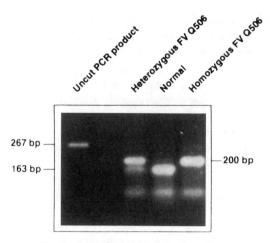

2% agarose gel of restriction products

Figure 2.3. Genomic DNA is amplified by the polymerase chain reaction using primers that span codon 506 of the factor V gene. The mutant factor V gene (A → G position 1691) results in a new *Mnl* I 200 base pair (bp) restriction fragment. The resulting gene product has a single amino acid substitution—glutamine (Q) for arginine (R)—that renders the molecule resistant to cleavage by APC. (Reproduced by permission from the American Heart Association, Inc., from Catto A, Carter A, Ireland H, et al. Factor V Leiden gene mutation and thrombin generation in relation to the development of acute stroke. Arterioscler Thromb Vasc Biol 1995;15:783–785.)

methods, all of which use extraction of whole blood DNA with amplification (using the *polymerase chain reaction*, PCR) of a small piece of the factor V gene containing the point mutation. Because the point mutation serendipitously eradicates a recognition sequence for the restriction enzyme *Mnl* I (which cleaves a specific nucleotide sequence in double-stranded DNA that is lost in APC resistance), the mutation in amplified DNA can be identified by a unique band pattern (reflecting different sized products) when *Mnl* I–digested DNA is size-separated by agarose gel electrophoresis. This technique can also identify the heterozygous or carrier state, which demonstrates a third band pattern in which all bands (derived from both normal and mutant DNA) are present in a single lane (Fig. 2.3).

Hyperhomocystinemia represents another example of the importance of translational research. Because homozygous cystathionine β-synthase deficiency, an inherited disease designated *homocystinuria*, is associated with venous thrombosis and premature atherosclerosis, a relationship was established between elevated blood homocysteine levels and thrombophilia. This relationship has been investigated extensively within the past few years, and it is clear that moderate hyperhomocystinemia is associated with a twofold to threefold increased risk of developing early-onset arterial and venous thromboses. The diagnosis of hyperhomocystinemia is made by measuring plasma homocysteine levels using high-performance liquid chromatography. Total plasma homocysteine levels are obtained following chemical treatment of plasma to release homocysteine bound to plasma proteins through a tight disulfide bond. What this means in practical terms is that a reliable reference laboratory is needed before a workup for hyperhomocystinemia is initiated. The range of normal versus abnormal plasma homocysteine levels overlaps somewhat, and the diagnostic workup perhaps can be made more predictive when homocysteine levels are measured 8 hours following an oral load of methionine (0.1 g/kg in 200 mL of fruit juice). Homocysteine levels increase in plasma after methionine ingestion because methionine is converted to homocysteine via metabolic pathways that normally conclude with the generation of cysteine. When the conversion is disrupted by a deficiency of the enzyme cystathionine β-synthase, homocysteine levels rise greatly. The pathophysiology and clinical aspects of hyperhomocystinemia are discussed further in Chapter 10.

Prothrombin G20210A is a common inherited mutation (guanine → adenine) in the non-coding 3′ region of the prothrombin gene found in about 2% of the Caucasian U.S. population. It causes levels of prothrombin (factor II) to increase to 115% to 130%, and it is diagnosed by a PCR-based assay of whole blood DNA.

Tests for **protein S, protein C, and antithrombin III deficiencies** are of two types: functional and immunological. The functional tests are relatively complicated and subject to alteration by exogenous factors (such as anticoagulation). Protein C or S activity should not be measured when a patient is taking warfarin (which inhibits protein S and protein C synthesis, as well as the synthesis of factors II, VII, IX, and X). Antithrombin III activity should not be measured when a patient is receiving heparin (which binds to antithrombin III and affects its in vitro activity). A normogram shows how warfarin affects the functional activities of proteins C and S (Table 2.3). There are many different types of immunological assays for the quantity of protein (antigen level). These are often done in conjunction with functional assays because of the theoretical concern that an immunologically unrecognizable mutation in the anticoagulant protein could affect function; this has been demonstrated with antithrombin III and protein C, but not protein S.

A **dysplasminogenemia** is associated with clinical thrombophilia. Laboratory studies typically reveal a normal antigenic level of plasma plasminogen with decreased functional activity. A deficiency of **heparin cofactor II**, which functions similarly to antithrombin III (see Chapter 5), leads to thrombophilia. Functional activity measurements are confounded by antithrombin III activity, and thus most functional assays require a step for removing antithrombin III. This removal step is the point where test variability arises. Reliable assays for either heparin cofactor II activity or antigen are not routinely available in most clinical laboratories, so studies must be sent to commercial reference laboratories or to the laboratory of a researcher willing to ensure proper control experiments. **Dysfibrinogenemias** usually cause bleeding. They are a rare cause of thrombophilia. Thrombophilia develops when the cleaved abnormal fibrinogen molecule is incorporated into insoluble fibrin, rendering the fibrin clot relatively

Table 2.3   The effects of anticoagulant therapy on the assay values of protein C and protein S, and factors II, IX, and X in patients with heterozygous protein C and S deficiencies and in nondeficient patients

	PROTEIN C (IU/dL)		PROTEIN S (U/dL)		FACTOR II (U/dL)		FACTOR IX (IU/dL)		FACTOR X (U/dL)	
	C	Ag	C	Ag	C	Ag	C	Ag	C	Ag
No anticoagulation										
Nondeficient	95	98	101	106	94	97	98	105	96	98
Protein C deficient	45	50	100	105	95	97	96	99	96	102
Protein S deficient	93	97	37	56	93	99	101	103	98	103
INR 2.0–2.5										
Nondeficient	40	54	65	87	44	63	55	61	42	44
Protein C deficient	26	29	64	86	46	64	52	60	43	46
Protein S deficient	40	55	28	50	45	62	51	59	42	45
INR 2.5–3.5										
Nondeficient	34	43	50	70	28	55	38	54	29	42
Protein C deficient	18	22	54	68	27	51	37	50	28	42
Protein S deficient	35	40	24	40	28	53	37	51	27	40
INR 3.5–4.5										
Nondeficient	22	39	43	66	23	47	29	46	24	38
Protein C deficient	11	16	44	65	24	44	27	49	23	37
Protein S deficient	23	36	19	33	22	48	26	47	24	37

Ag, antigenic level; C, coagulant activity; INR, international normalized ratio.

Reproduced with permission from Loscalzo J, Schafer AI, eds. Thrombosis and hemorrhage. 2nd ed. Philadelphia: Lippincott Williams & Wilkins, 1998:483. Copyright © 1998, Lippincott Williams & Wilkins Co.

resistant to fibrinolysis with plasmin. In these cases, the antigenic quantity of fibrinogen is normal, while the activity measured in a thrombin time assay can be either normal or decreased. Measurement of the plasmin sensitivity of a fibrin clot from a patient who is suspected of having this condition is performed only in a few research laboratories.

Annotated Bibliography

1. Bockenstedt PL. Laboratory methods in hemostasis. In: Loscalzo J, Schafer AI, eds. Thrombosis and hemorrhage. 2nd ed. Philadelphia: Lippincott Williams & Wilkins, 1998:517–582.

   This is a comprehensive, and comprehensible, summary of current clinical laboratory methods applied to the diagnosis of bleeding and clotting problems.

2. Lind SE. The bleeding time does not predict surgical bleeding. Blood 1991;77:2547–2552.

   An effectively dogmatic review assailing the routine use of screening bleeding times during a preoperative evaluation. When would you do a bleeding time preoperatively? Only in patients with a clear-cut personal or family history of bleeding (in my opinion). In the opinion of Lind, the usefulness of the preoperative bleeding time is generally unproven, but worthy of study in patients with uremia, aspirin ingestion, planned microvascular procedures, and a history of bleeding.

3. Fermo I, Vigano' D'Angelo S, Paroni R, Mazzola G, Calori G, D'Angelo A. Prevalence of moderate hyperhomocysteinemia in patients with early-onset venous and arterial occlusive disease. Ann Intern Med 1995;123:747–753.

   This is an important paper for at least two reasons: it describes the prevalence of elevated plasma homocysteine levels in patients less than 45 years old with diseases of the arterial and venous circuits (19.2% and 13.1%, respectively), and it begins to develop some standardization of laboratory tests required to make predictions about the significance of plasma homocysteine levels under basal and loaded conditions.

3

An Overview of Thrombotic Disorders and Their Treatment

The pathogenesis of thrombosis can be organized conceptually by considering it an imbalance between those components of Virchow's triad that are antithrombotic and those components of Virchow's triad that are prothrombotic (see Chapter 1). Any individual pathogenetic factor, or combination of pathogenetic factors, that decreases antithrombotic processes and/or increases prothrombotic processes can lead to thrombosis (Fig. 3.1). In practice, thromboses usually involve either the venous circulation or the arterial circulation, although there are examples of thrombotic disorders that involve both veins and arteries (e.g., antiphospholipid antibodies) and those in which venous thromboembolism crosses over to the aorta through an intracardiac shunt (e.g., paradoxical embolism).

Thrombotic Disorders Are the Most Common Diseases Affecting Americans

The common thrombotic disorders seen by physicians in many clinical settings are thrombosis in the deep veins of the legs associated with surgery, hospitalization, or debilitating chronic illnesses, and thrombosis due to chronic atherosclerotic arterial diseases (particularly of the coronary, carotid, and large peripheral arteries). Together, these conditions affect tens of millions, and kill several million persons every year in the United States. All physicians should be familiar with their pathophysiology and treatment.

Thrombotic Disorders Are Frequently Misunderstood

The hypercoagulable states are often considered when investigating patients with thrombosis, yet they account for relatively few patients overall. Hypercoagulable states usually are associated with venous thrombosis. There remains significant misunderstanding about evaluating patients for hypercoagulability

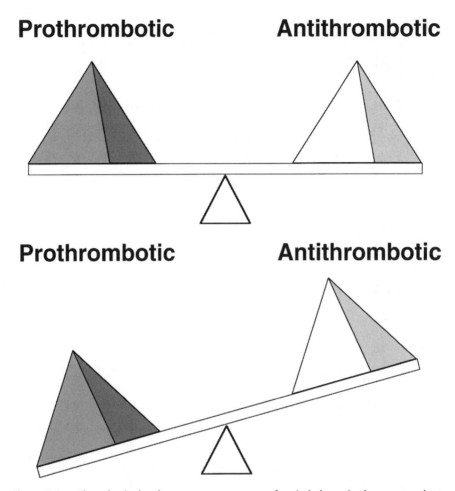

Figure 3.1. Thrombosis develops as a consequence of an imbalance in the procoagulant and anticoagulant factors operating within Virchow's triad. There may be increased procoagulant function and/or decreased anticoagulant function involving, individually or in combination, the blood, the vessel wall, and blood flow.

(i.e., when and how to "work up" patients for this condition). Such misunderstanding of the hypercoagulable states has decreased in the past few years, and new focus on laboratory testing and treatment options has (for once) simultaneously simplified and strengthened the current approach to thrombophilic patients (see Chapter 10).

Rare Thrombotic Disorders Are Important

There are many other interesting and clinically important thrombotic disorders that lead to nonatheromatous arterial thrombosis, such as the antiphospholipid antibody syndrome (Chapter 9), thrombotic thrombocytopenic purpura (Chapter 12), and heparin-induced thrombocytopenia with thrombosis (Chapter 14). Although they are relatively uncommon in general medical or surgical practices, all physicians should expect to encounter them at some time during their careers. Furthermore, each provides an elegant clinical example of how specific pathogenetic factors lead to a prothrombotic imbalance in Virchow's triad. Our understanding of the pathogenesis of rare thrombotic disorders has been the source for the flow of ideas and reagents that has moved the standard of care for *all* patients with coagulation disorders great distances during the past decade.

4

Venous Thromboembolism

Venous thromboembolism (VTE) is extremely common in sick people. Deep venous thrombosis (DVT) and pulmonary embolism (PE) need to be considered as a single disease process in which red thrombi originating in the leg veins become dislodged and travel through the right heart into the pulmonary artery. The natural history of DVT involves progression to PE in at least 50% of cases and at least 70% of PEs are associated with a measurable DVT. Recent estimates indicate that symptomatic DVT develops in about 600,000 and PE in 630,000 persons annually in the United States (1). These numbers undoubtedly under-represent the total number of patients with DVT and PE, as most patients are asymptomatic.

To put the scope of the problem in perspective, Weinmann and Salzman (1) considered the natural history in a population of patients:

At least 30 cases of DVT identifiable by phlebography can be expected among 100 patients who have undergone general surgical operations of moderate severity if they are not given perioperative antithrombotic prophylaxis. Most postoperative thrombi arise in the calves . . . but in at least 20 percent of patients who have undergone general surgical procedures and 40 to 50 percent of patients with skeletal trauma, thrombi can originate in more proximal veins. Isolated calf thrombi are often asymptomatic. If untreated 20 to 30 percent may extend into the larger more proximal veins, an event that accounts for most clinically important pulmonary emboli and virtually all fatal ones. Among these 100 patients, four cases of pulmonary emboli will be recognized; one or two may be fatal. Many more patients will have silent, clinically unrecognized pulmonary emboli.

Now consider that, according to the American Hospital Association, in 1991 to 1992 there were approximately 33,500,000 admissions to 6500 U.S. hospitals, including admissions for 24 million operations. Assuming (conservatively) that 20 million U.S. patients were at risk for venous thromboembolism during this time, and that only 50% of these patients were given adequate prophylaxis (based on information from the Mayo Clinic [2]), at least 3 million patients had proximal DVT and two-thirds went unrecognized and untreated. Thus, 2 million individuals represent the discrepancy between patients who are at risk but untreated and patients who have been diagnosed. Approximately 40% of the 2 million patients with unrecognized proximal DVT will have asymptomatic PE. Of the 800,000 patients with silent PE, at least 10% (80,000) cases will be fatal and remain unrecognized unless the patient undergoes a postmortem examination (3). At the Mayo Clinic, one-half of fatal PEs were only discovered at autopsy, so it is reasonable to assume that each year many of the U.S. patients whose certified cause is PE (at least 100,000) died of a disease process completely unrecognized or unsuspected antemortem (2).

Nor can outpatients be overlooked; they are not necessarily protected by the simple fact that they are *not* hospitalized. They suffer the same risk factors as hospitalized patients. Although no epidemiological data are available about symptomatic or asymptomatic venous thromboembolism in outpatients, one must consider that their risk is *at least equal* to that of hospitalized patients suffering from comparable illnesses.

It is extremely difficult to determine through a bedside examination which patients have a DVT or a PE, and there are no readily available screening studies. The classic findings of a tender and swollen calf, with venous distension and pain on foot dorsiflexion (Homans' sign), occur in less than one-half of patients with DVT. Similarly, at least one-half of patients with PE, including those who will have fatal PE, are asymptomatic.

As a first step in dealing with the difficulty in diagnosis, it is imperative to *employ appropriate prophylactic measures in every patient you see in a clinic, during an office visit, on a hospital ward, or at home.* The second step is to *bring to every patient you see a high index of suspicion for venous thromboembolic diseases.*

Prevention

Prevention is the first and most important step in dealing with venous thromboembolism. Prevention can be accomplished by remaining vigilant for risk factors in *every* patient, and by using prophylaxis in every case in which it is appropriate. Table 4.1 lists the risk factors and prophylactic measures for hospitalized patients. In cases of surgery, the prophylactic antithrombotic agent is started within 24 hours of the operation, continued for 7 to 10 days, and stopped a day or two after the patient is fully ambulatory. In other situations when prophylaxis is indicated, it is usually started when the risk of hemorrhage plateaus and is continued until the thrombotic risk passes. Among symptomatic outpatients with DVT, the major risk factors appear to be immobilization, trauma, and recent surgery; prophylaxis should be used routinely among these patients. One should also consider using long-term prophylaxis among all outpatients with cancer and heart failure, even if they are relatively mobile (4).

Certain types of high-risk patients do better on a prophylactic regimen other than heparin (5000 U subcutaneously, twice a day). Currently, according to the

Table 4.1   Risk of venous thrombosis and recommended prophylaxis

EVENT OR CONDITION	LOW RISK	MODERATE RISK[a]	HIGH RISK[a]
General surgery	Age < 40 years; duration of operation < 60 minutes	Age > 40 years; duration of operation > 60 minutes	Age > 40 years; duration of operation > 60 minutes; and additional risk factors: previous deep-vein thrombosis or pulmonary emboli or extensive tumor
Orthopedic surgery	—	—	Elective hip or knee arthroplasty
Trauma	—	—	Extensive soft tissue injury; major fractures; multiple trauma
Medical conditions	Pregnancy	Myocardial infarction; congestive heart failure; postpartum period, especially with previous deep-vein thrombosis or pulmonary emboli	Stroke
Incidence of thromboembolic events without prophylaxis (%)			
• Distal deep-vein thrombosis—calf veins	2	10–40	40–80
• Proximal deep-vein thrombosis—pelvis, thigh, and popliteal veins	0.4	2–8	10–20
• Symptomatic pulmonary emboli	0.2	1–8	5–10
• Fatal pulmonary emboli	0.002	0.1–0.4	1–5
Recommended prophylaxis	Graduated compression stockings and early ambulation	Heparin (5000 U, subcutaneously, twice daily), low-molecular-weight heparin or external pneumatic compression, or intravenous dextran	Heparin (5000 U, subcutaneously, three times daily), low-molecular-weight heparin, external pneumatic compression, intravenous dextran, warfarin (adjusted dose), vena caval interruption, or percutaneous insertion of intracaval filters

[a] The risk is increased by the following factors: older age, obesity, prolonged bed rest, varicose veins, and estrogen treatment.
Reprinted by permission of the New England Journal of Medicine, from Weinmann EE, Salzman EW. Deep-vein thrombosis. N Engl J Med 1994;331:1630–1641.

recommendations of the American Heart Association and the American Association of Chest Physicians, either adjusted-dose unfractionated heparin, low-dose warfarin (aiming for an International Normalized Ratio [INR] of 2.0; see Chapter 5), or fixed low-molecular-weight heparin (LMWH; see Chapter 5) is superior to unfractionated heparin administered as 5000 U subcutaneously, twice a day to prevent venous thromboembolism in patients undergoing orthopedic surgery, or in patients with a history of recurrent thrombosis (5). LMWH is probably the treatment of choice for patients who are undergoing hip or knee replacement surgery, and for patients with spinal cord injury. The best preventive program for neurosurgical patients is a single daily subcutaneous injection of the LMWH enoxaparin (40 mg) combined with compression stockings (6). Note that no LMWH preparation has yet been approved by the U.S. Food and Drug Administration for use in spinal cord injury or neurosurgical patients, despite ample data that these drugs have a superior therapeutic index. Chronic debilitated cancer patients should be treated with long-term warfarin targeting an INR of 2.0.

A reasonable question at this time is why prophylaxis is not administered to every sick person, regardless of outpatient or inpatient status. In fact, prophylaxis *should* be given to all sick patients, but prophylaxis in low-risk patients involves nonpharmacologic measures such as graduated compression stockings and forced ambulation. In this population, pharmacologic prophylaxis cannot be currently recommended because its cost-effectiveness and risk-benefit ratios have not been proven to be favorable.

In high-risk patients anticoagulant therapy is cost-effective, although the most clearly cost-effective regimen has yet to emerge. It costs about $12 per day for 5000 U of heparin, administered subcutaneously twice a day: $6 for the drug, and $6 cost for the administration. Enoxaparin (Lovenox) costs about $29 per day for 30 mg administered subcutaneously twice a day: $23 for the drug, and $6 for the administration. Although the retail cost for warfarin is much less than either of the heparin preparations, the cost of laboratory monitoring (maintaining an international normalized ratio [INR] of 2.0) inevitably makes it at least as expensive.

As far as the medical risks of prophylaxis, bleeding is the primary concern. The rate of bleeding among patients receiving unfractionated heparin (5000 U, subcutaneously, twice a day) is about 5% to 10%, with 1% to 2% being "major bleeding" (defined as a fall of Hgb > 2 g/dL, or retroperitoneal or intracranial bleeding). Bleeding complications from prophylactic LMWH are about one-half less frequent than from unfractionated heparin. Both unfractionated heparin and LMWH are associated with the development of heparin-associated thrombocytopenia, although it has been established that this condition is less likely to occur with LMWH than with standard heparin (see Chapter 5). Long-term administration of all heparin preparations leads to osteoporosis. Warfarin therapy with a target INR of 2.0–2.5 leads to bleeding in approximately 5% of patients; there are generally fewer bleeding complications with carefully monitored warfarin therapy (INR = 2.0) than with any heparin preparation.

Table 4.2 Results of the international multicenter trial of prevention of postoperative venous thromboembolism with low-dose heparin

	CONTROL GROUP[a]	HEPARIN GROUP[b]	*P*
Fatal pulmonary emboli	16 of 2076 (0.8%)	2 of 2045 (0.1%)	<.005
Clinically diagnosed pulmonary emboli	24 of 2076 (1.2%)	8 of 2075 (0.4%)	<.01
Symptomatic DVT (confirmed by venography)	32 of 2076 (1.5%)	11 of 2075 (0.5%)	<.005
Venous thrombosis by RFUT	164 of 667 (25%)	48 of 625 (8%)	<.005

Abbreviations: DVT = deep-vein thrombosis; RFUT = radioactive fibrinogen uptake test.

[a] No prophylaxis.

[b] Calcium heparin, 5000 U subcutaneously 2 hours before surgery and every 8 hours for 7 days. Reproduced with permission from Loscalzo J, Schafer AI, eds. Thrombosis and hemorrhage. 2nd ed. Philadelphia: Lippincott Williams & Wilkins, 1998. Copyright © 1998, Lippincott Williams & Wilkins Co.

The dividends from assessing risk and implementing prophylaxis are excellent. Table 4.2 shows the effectiveness of prophylactic measures in general surgical patients treated with heparin (5000 U subcutaneously, twice a day). The study from which these data are derived was published in 1975. More recent data using contrast venography to assess the effectiveness of DVT prophylaxis in patients undergoing hip and knee replacement demonstrate that warfarin (adjusted to maintain an INR of 2.0) or LMWH reduces the development of DVT by at least 50%, with LMWH showing a slight advantage in terms of efficacy and a slight disadvantage in terms of toxicity (bleeding) (7,8). These studies also show that at least one-third of the treated patients develop a DVT, with about 7% overall getting a high-risk proximal DVT. These results emphasize that one cannot let one's guard down simply because preventive measures have been implemented, as prophylaxis alone fails to prevent proximal DVT in a significant percentage of patients. This leads to the obvious questions: How does one diagnose venous thromboembolism, and how does one use the diagnostic information?

Diagnosis of DVT and PE

DVT and PE should be considered in any patient at risk who has not been given adequate prophylaxis, and those who have received prophylaxis should be watched warily. Certainly all orthopedic, cancer, surgical, and/or bed-bound medical patients must be considered to be at *constant high risk*. Daily leg examinations must be performed, looking not only for Homans' sign, but also for lower extremity edema or calf diameter asymmetry, which develops in about 25% of DVT patients. Most experts agree that the bedside examination is not a reliable predictor of a positive or negative venogram, so diagnostic testing should be applied to all patients suspected of having a DVT. A "Chinese menu" approach to the bedside diagnosis of DVT has been proposed but not rigorously validated (9). The criteria used to establish a high prevenogram probability of DVT in this model can be applied to the examination of all patients and might be used to guide the diagnostic evaluation, but they should not be used to rule definitively on a DVT or to direct therapeutic interventions (Table 4.3).

The subtle but common bedside manifestations of PE—such as dyspnea and tachypnea (in at least 75%), tachycardia (50%), rales (40%), temperature over 37.8°C (30%), and syncope (25%)—should also be looked for. Classic findings

Table 4.3   Clinical model for predicting pretest (venography) probability for deep-vein thrombosis

Checklist

Major points
Active cancer (treatment ongoing or within previous 6 months or palliative)
Paralysis, paresis, or recent plaster immobilization of the lower extremities
Recently bedridden over 3 days and/or major surgery within 4 weeks
Localized tenderness along the distribution of the deep venous system
Thigh and calf swollen (should be measured)
Calf swelling 3 cm more than symptomless side (measured 10 cm below tibial tuberosity)
Strong family history of DVT (≥2 first-degree relatives with history of DVT)

Minor points
History of recent trauma (≥60 days) to the symptomatic leg
Pitting edema; symptomatic leg only
Dilated superficial veins (non-varicose) in symptomatic leg only
Hospitalization within previous 6 months
Erythema

Clinical probability
High
    ≥3 major points and no alternative diagnosis
    ≥2 major points and ≥2 minor points + no alternative diagnosis
Low
    1 major point + ≥2 minor points + has an alternative diagnosis
    1 major point + ≥1 minor point + no alternative diagnosis
    0 major points + ≥3 minor points + has an alternative diagnosis
    0 major points + ≥2 minor points + no alternative diagnosis
Moderate
    All other combinations

Active cancer did not include non-melanomatous skin cancer; deep-vein tenderness had to be elicited in either the calf or thigh in the anatomical distribution of the deep venous system.

Reproduced by permission from Wells PS, Hirsh J, Anderson DR, et al. Accuracy of clinical assessment of deep-vein thrombosis. Lancet 1995;345:1326–1330.

of pulmonary infarction (dyspnea, pleuritic chest pain, and hemoptysis) are found in less than 10% of all PE patients (Table 4.4). In fact, the presence of these symptoms should alert the physician to the possibility of massive PE, where rapid diagnosis can reap the benefits of thrombolytic therapy. In every

Table 4.4 Clinical symptoms and signs in 92 patients with fatal pulmonary embolism

	PATIENTS	
FINDING	No.	%
Symptom		
Dyspnea	54	59
Syncope	25	27
Altered mental state	18	20
Apprehension	16	17
Chest pain (not pleuritic)	9	10
Sweatiness	8	9
Pleuritic pain	7	8
Cough	3	3
Hemoptysis	3	3
None other than sudden arrest	7	8
Sign		
Respiratory rate ≥16/min	61	66
Tachycardia (HR > 100 beats/min)	50	54
Rales	39	42
Temperature > 37.8°C	28	30
Lower extremity edema	24	26
Sudden hypotension	18	20
Cyanosis	11	12
Gallop rhythm	9	10
Diaphoresis	9	10
Phlebitis	6	7
Increased S_2P	2	2
None other than sudden arrest	4	4

Not all symptoms and signs were acute in onset. Including patients on ventilators (4), unresponsive or sedated (4), in a coma (2), or with sudden arrest as the only acute "symptom" (24), 32 of the 92 patients (35%) were judged on the basis of clinical records to have been unable to describe new symptoms to their physician.

Abbreviations: HR = heart rate; S_2P = pulmonic component of the second heart sound.

Reproduced by permission from Morgenthaler TI, Ryu JH. Clinical characteristics of fatal pulmonary embolism in a referral hospital. Mayo Clin Proc 1995;70:417–424.

case, a quick workup is indicated because treatment must be initiated as early as possible within the course of the thrombosis. When a PE is fatal, the death usually occurs rapidly—within a day of the development of symptoms.

The diagnosis of DVT and PE can be made by following the algorithms shown in Figure 4.1. As seen in Table 4.5, every test is quite sensitive in symptomatic patients, but noninvasive testing is generally insensitive for asymptomatic patients. In asymptomatic patients, going directly to contrast venography is therefore reasonable. Contrast venography is the standard against which all other diagnostic tests are compared. It is not done in every patient because it can be an uncomfortable procedure, and it is associated with a 2% to 3% risk of causing DVT.

Diagnostic Evaluation of DVT

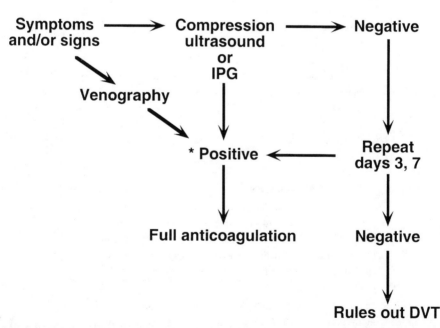

A

Figure 4.1.   (A) Diagnostic evaluation of DVT. (B) Diagnostic evaluation of PE. (*If the thrombus is limited to the calf, anticoagulation can be held if serial examination with ultrasound or IPG fails to show proximal propagation over 14 days.)

Diagnostic Evaluation of PE

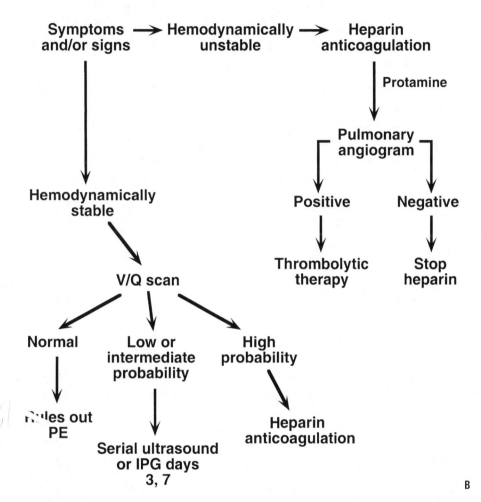

Figure 4.1.　**Continued.**

Table 4.6, which shows some results of comparing V/Q scans with pulmonary angiography, illustrates four important points: 1) a low-probability lung scan does not rule out PE; 2) a high-probability lung scan is a false-positive result in up to one-third of patients; 3) almost one-half of all patients with PE do *not* have a high probability V/Q scan; and 4) a normal study is a reliable way to rule out PE in 99% of patients. Therefore, in patients where the clinical suspicion of PE is high, a low-probability V/Q scan must be followed up by evaluating patients for DVT with the use of serial doppler ultrasound or

Table 4.5   Tests used in the diagnosis of deep-vein thrombosis

TEST	SYMPTOMATIC DEEP-VEIN THROMBOSIS[a]		ASYMPTOMATIC DEEP-VEIN THROMBOSIS[b]		ANATOMICAL AREA	COMMENT
	Sensitivity (%)	Specificity (%)	Sensitivity (%)	Specificity (%)		
Phlebography	Standard for comparison		Standard for comparison		Pelvis, thigh, popliteal area, calf	Invasive; provides equivocal results in cases of recurrent deep-vein thrombosis; not easily repeated
Impedance plethysmography	92[c]	95	22	98	Thigh, popliteal area	For provisional diagnosis of primary or recurrent proximal deep-vein thrombosis; insensitive to calf thrombi and to nonocclusive proximal thrombi
Ultrasonography Real-time B-mode or duplex	97	97	59	98	Thigh, popliteal area	Most sensitive confirmatory test for symptomatic deep-vein thrombosis
Doppler flow velocity	88	88	—	—	Thigh, popliteal area	Can be used on limbs in traction or plaster; interpretation is subjective, requires skill
Magnetic resonance venography[d]	96	100	—	—	Inferior vena cava, pelvis, thigh	Can distinguish between acute and chronic occlusion; can identify associated abnormalities; noninvasive; expensive; limited availability

Note: No data on [^{125}I]-labeled fibrinogen scanning were included, as the test is no longer available.
[a] Testing is mostly used to verify clinical suspicion of deep-vein thrombosis.
[b] Testing is mostly used to screen high-risk patients.
[c] Recent studies have reported lower sensitivity.
[d] Magnetic resonance venography has only been evaluated in small clinical trials.

Reprinted by permission of the New England Journal of Medicine, from Weinmann EE, Salzman EW. Deep-vein thrombosis. N Engl J Med

Table 4.6   Ventilation-perfusion lung scan results according to the presence or absence of pulmonary embolism (by arteriography)

SCAN RESULT	NUMBER OF PATIENTS	PULMONARY EMBOLISM	NO PULMONARY EMBOLISM
High probability	178	108	70
Intermediate probability	127	20	107
Low probability	261	64	197
Normal	400	4	396

Reproduced by permission from Hull RD, Raskob GE. Low-probability lung scan findings: a need for change. Ann Intern Med 1991;114:142–143.

impedence plethysmography evaluations. This is based on data that about 70% of PEs will have synchronous DVT.

How does one deal with the false-positive high-probability results of a V/Q scan? Most experts recommend full treatment for these patients. If there are confounding clinical conditions that make the need for a precise diagnosis essential (i.e., ongoing hemorrhage, recent intracranial surgery, hemorrhagic stroke, or a history of heparin-associated thrombocytopenia), a pulmonary angiogram should be done. In fact, the simplicity and safety of pulmonary angiography have been improved, and it should be used in any case where clinical/laboratory ambiguities exist (10).

In an effort to streamline the diagnosis of venous thromboembolism, the measurement of plasma levels of D-dimers has been extensively investigated. D-dimers are products of plasmin-mediated digestion of cross-linked fibrin, and their levels are elevated in states of increased coagulation such as DVT and PE. Current data indicate that D-dimers are not useful in the diagnosis of PE (either ruling them in or ruling them out), and probably should not be used to screen for PE (10,11). D-dimers may be more useful for ruling out DVT, and early reports describe a good sensitivity of the D-dimer measurement in *symptomatic patients when it is combined with a clinical score* (similar to Table 4.3). In two studies, the absence of D-dimers among patients with a low-risk clinical score proved to be a very reliable way to rule out DVT (12,13). Time will tell exactly how D-dimer measurements are to be used. For now, D-dimer testing should be considered investigative.

Treatment of DVT and PE with Anticoagulants

The treatment options in the United States for patients with acute DVT and PE are currently heparin, streptokinase, urokinase, and tPA; LMWH and the heparinoid danaparoid are also available for treating acute VTE, although not all products have been FDA-approved for this indication (14–18) (Chapter 5). Warfarin is the only oral anticoagulant routinely used for maintenance therapy. Table 4.7 gives the standard treatment for DVT and PE in the United States. Table 4.8 shows an effective alternative treatment plan based on a

Table 4.7   Standard treatment of venous thromboembolism with unfractionated intravenous heparin and oral warfarin

Initiate therapy with heparin

1. Administer heparin, 5000 U intravenously, and start an infusion of 1200 U/hour.
2. Check aPTT after 4 to 6 hours and adjust infusion to prolong aPTT to 1.5–2.5 times control.

   (*Alternative*) Administer heparin subcutaneously every 12 hours beginning with an initial dose of 18,000 U. Check aPTT after 4 hours and adjust subsequent dose to prolong aPTT to 1.5–2.5 times control.

Maintenance anticoagulation

Oral anticoagulants

1. Begin warfarin, 5 mg, during first hospital day.
2. Check PT daily.
3. Adjust dose to achieve INR of 2.0–3.0.
4. Discontinue heparin after minimum of 5 days when INR reaches 2.0 for two consecutive days.
5. Continue warfarin as outpatient for 6 months.

Heparin

1. Administer heparin subcutaneously every 12 hours in a dose to prolong the mid-interval aPTT to 1.5 times control.

aPTT = activated partial thromboplastin time; INR = international normalized ratio; PT = prothrombin time.

Reproduced with permission from Loscalzo J, Schafer AI, eds. Thrombosis and hemorrhage. 2nd ed. Philadelphia: Lippincott Williams & Wilkins, 1998. Copyright ©1998, Lippincott Williams & Wilkins Co.

patient's weight. Subcutaneous heparin is as effective as infused heparin as long as the therapeutic activated partial thromboplastin time (aPTT) is achieved rapidly and maintained at 1.5 to 2.5 times the control. It is essential that a therapeutic aPTT be achieved within the first 24 hours of treatment to minimize the chances of thromboembolism (Table 4.9). Table 4.10 suggests a strategy for accomplishing this end point. The use of a LMWH heparin (e.g., 1 mg/kg of enoxaparin, subcutaneously, every 12 hours) may soon usurp the use of unfractionated heparin therapy during the induction phase of treatment, and currently two preparations are approved for such use: enoxaparin and tinzaparin (16–18). Two recent reports document that outpatient treatment of DVT with LMWH is both safe and effective, and it is likely that this will become routine management of selected patients (19,20).

Maintenance treatment is generally continued for at least 6 months; treatment for 6 weeks (21) or 3 months (22) is clearly inadequate. For maintenance therapy, subcutaneous heparin administered three times per day to maintain the aPTT at 1.5 times the control aPTT (4 hours after the preceding dose) is as efficacious as warfarin. The overall mortality for patients with venous thromboembolism treated conventionally with heparin followed by 6 months of warfarin is about 4% after 2 years, with a recurrence rate of over 10% after

Table 4.8 A sample weight-based heparin order sheet

Heparin Order Sheet
(All blanks must be filled in by physician)

1. Make calculations using total body weight: _____ kg.
2. BOLUS HEPARIN, 80 units/kg = _____ units IV
3. IV HEPARIN infusion, 18 units/kg·h = _____ units/h (20,000 units heparin in 500 mL of D5W, 40 units per mL)
4. WARFARIN _____ mg. PO QD to start on second day of heparin
5. LABORATORY: APTT, PT, CBC now
   CBC with platelet count Q 3 days
   STAT APTT 6 hours after heparin bolus
   PT Q day (start on third day of heparin)
6. ADJUST heparin infusion based on sliding scale below:

PTT < 35	80 unit s/kg bolus = _____ units
	increase drip 4 units/kg·h = _____ units/h
PTT 35 to 45	40 unit s/kg bolus = _____ units
	increase drip 2 units/kg·h = _____ units/h
PTT 46 to 70	No change
PTT 71 to 90	reduce drip 2 units/kg·h = _____ units/h
PTT > 90	hold heparin for 1 h,
	reduce drip 3 units/kg·h = _____ units/h

7. Order a PTT 6 hours after any dosage change, adjusting heparin infusion by the sliding scale until PTT is therapeutic (46 to 70 seconds). When 2 consecutive PTTs are therapeutic, order PTT (and re-adjust heparin drip as needed) every 24 hours.

Please make changes as promptly as possible and round off doses to the nearest mL/h (nearest 40 units per hour).

Signed: _____ Date: _____

A sample weight-based heparin order sheet.

Reproduced by permission from Raschke RA, Reilly BM, Guidry JR, et al. The weight-based heparin dosing nomogram compared with a "standard care" nomogram. A randomized controlled trial. Ann Intern Med 1993;119:874–881. © American College of Physicians, 1993.

2 years. The rate of recurrence appears to be highest during the first 6 months after diagnosis. After this period the recurrence rate declines, although it never becomes zero because of the presence of chronically damaged valves in the deep veins of the affected legs. Among a group of patients with a first symptomatic

Table 4.9   It is imperative to achieve a therapeutic aPTT within the first 24 hours of beginning a heparin infusion

	FREQUENCY OF RECURRENT VENOUS THROMBOEMBOLISM (NO. OF PATIENTS)		
TREATMENT GROUP	aPTT Response < Lower Limit[a]	aPTT Response ≥ Lower Limit[a]	P VALUE
Subcutaneous	10 of 36 (27.8)	1 of 21 (4.8)	.041
Intravenous	3 of 17 (17.6)	0 of 41	.022
All patients[b]	13 of 53 (24.5)	1 of 62 (1.6)	<.001

[a] The figures in parentheses are percentages.

[b] The relative risk of recurrent venous thromboembolism was 15 times higher in patients with an aPTT response below the lower limit (1.5 times control) of the prescribed range for 24 hours or more from the start of therapy than in patients with an aPTT response at or above the lower limit.

Reproduced with permission from Loscalzo J, Schafer AI, eds. Thrombosis and hemorrhage. 2nd ed. Philadelphia: Lippincott Williams & Wilkins, 1998. Copyright ©1998, Lippincott Williams & Wilkins Co.

Table 4.10   Standard approach to optimize aPTT response

Initial dose	5000 unit bolus then 1000 U/hour
aPTT < 35s	5000 unit bolus and increase infusion by 200 U/hour
aPTT 35–45s	2500 unit bolus and increase infusion by 100 U/hour
aPTT 46–70s	No change
aPTT 71–90s	Decrease rate by 100 U/hour
aPTT > 90s	Hold infusion for 1 hour, then decrease rate by 200 U/hour

Reproduced by permission from Raschke RA, Reilly BM, Guidry JR, et al. The weight-based heparin dosing nomogram compared with a "standard care" nomogram. A randomized controlled trial. Ann Intern Med 1993;119:874–881.

DVT, the risk of recurrence in the ipsilateral leg was 17.5% at 2 years, 25% at 5 years, and 30% at 8 years (23). Recent recommendations by the American Heart Association state that a recurrent ipsilateral DVT is unequivocally established only when there is a new filling defect observed by venography (24). Be warned that a clinical bedside diagnosis of ipsilateral recurrence of a DVT is usually wrong and that distinguishing the symptoms and signs of "post-phlebitic syndrome" from recurrent DVT at the bedside is impossible.

The post-phlebitic syndrome is an important risk factor for recurrent DVT (23). Besides being dangerous, it is also uncomfortable and expensive (the health care system will spend 75% of the cost of treating the acute DVT to manage the post-phlebitic syndrome) (25). Patients with acute DVT who wear compression stockings for a few weeks after diagnosis suffer fewer post-phlebitic problems; this simple trick to prevent a major long-term complication of DVT is recommended for all patients with acute proximal DVT (26).

The risk of bleeding over 6 months of treatment is related to the care with which the INR is maintained within the 2.0 to 3.0 range, or the mid-dose aPTT is kept at 1.5 times the control. When these are done, the risk of major bleeding is only 1%. When too much warfarin or heparin is given, the risk of major bleeding increases and there is a small (approximately 1%) chance of fatal bleeding. In a recent study comparing 24 versus 6 months of warfarin carefully maintained at an INR of 2.0–3.0, 3 of 79 patients (3.8%) assigned to warfarin had nonfatal major bleeding (two gastrointestinal and one genitourinary hemorrhages). None of the 83 patients assigned to placebo had bleeding.

The optimal duration of treatment has yet to be established. The risk for recurrence is highest in patients with an ongoing risk factor, such as a previous VTE, active cancer, or a hypercoagulable state (see Chapter 10). These types of patients probably should be considered for long-term warfarin anticoagulation; such a treatment will decrease the risk of recurrent VTE and increase the risk of bleeding, but probably will have no effect on overall mortality (27).

Thrombolytic Therapy

Thrombolytic therapy with streptokinase, urokinase, or tissue plasminogen activator (tPA) has been used to treat venous thromboembolism, and it is the treatment of choice for hemodynamically unstable PE. Table 4.11 suggests which patients are candidates for thrombolytic therapy, and Table 4.12 gives the dosages of three thrombolytic agents that are available in the United States for treating PE. Bleeding complications are generally greater with thrombolytic therapy: for tPA, approximately 45% with 14% major bleeding; for unfrac-

Table 4.11 **Relative indications and contraindications to thrombolytic therapy for patients with venous thromboembolism**

Treat those most likely to respond and benefit from thrombolytic therapy
- Deep-vein thrombosis: large, proximal thrombi with symptoms for less than 7 days
- Pulmonary embolism: massive or submassive embolism especially with hemodynamic compromise

Select patients to avoid bleeding complications
- Major contraindications
  1. Risk of intracranial bleeding: recent head trauma, or central nervous system surgery, history of stroke or subarachnoid bleed, intracranial metastatic disease
  2. Risk of major bleeding: active gastrointestinal or genitourinary bleeding, major surgery or trauma within 7 days
- Relative contraindications
  1. Remote history of gastrointestinal or genitourinary bleeding or peptic ulcer or other lesion with potential for bleeding, recent minor surgery or trauma, severe uncontrolled hypertension, coexisting hemostatic abnormalities

Reproduced with permission from Loscalzo J, Schafer AI, eds. Thrombosis and hemorrhage. 2nd ed. Philadelphia: Lippincott Williams & Wilkins, 1998. Copyright ©1998, Lippincott Williams & Wilkins Co.

Table 4.12   Thrombolytic therapies

Streptokinase

Dose	250,000 U intravenously over 15–20 minutes followed by a continuous infusion of 100,000 U/hour
Duration	12–24 hours for pulmonary embolism; 2–3 days or longer for deep-vein thrombosis
Advantages	Largest experience; inexpensive
Disadvantages	Occasional allergic reactions; low percentage of population has high-titer neutralizing antibodies

Urokinase

Dose	4400 U/kg intravenously over 15–20 minutes, followed by a constant infusion of 4400 U/kg per hour
Duration	12–24 hours for pulmonary embolism; 2–3 days or longer for deep-vein thrombosis
Advantages	Not antigenic
Disadvantages	More expensive than streptokinase

rt-PA (for pulmonary embolism only)

Dose	100 mg intravenously as a constant infusion over 2 hours
Duration	2 hours
Advantages	Not antigenic; short treatment duration
Disadvantages	Least experience; most expensive; pulmonary embolism only

rt-PA = recombinant tissue-type plasminogen activator.

Reproduced with permission from Loscalzo J, Schafer AI, eds. Thrombosis and hemorrhage. 2nd ed. Philadelphia: Lippincott Williams & Wilkins, 1998. Copyright ©1998, Lippincott Williams & Wilkins Co.

tionated heparin, approximately 20% with 3% major bleeding. The greatest risk of bleeding is at sites of angiogram catheter puncture. Streptokinase or urokinase are usually continued for 12 to 24 hours, and the patient is thereafter routinely anticoagulated with heparin.

There are no data that indicate that thrombolytic therapy decreases mortality among patients with venous thromboembolism, including PE associated with hemodynamic instability. Rather, by lysing the fibrin clot thrombolytics can improve clinical outcome. Table 4.13 shows that, in DVT, thrombolytics improve the reestablishment of vein patency and preserve valve function, thereby decreasing the likelihood of the post-phlebitic syndrome. Thrombolytics also improve the patency rate of the thrombosed pulmonary artery, thereby decreasing pulmonary artery pressures and improving both short-term and long-term lung functions. For these reasons, thrombolytic therapy is recommended for PE associated with hemodynamic stability.

Inferior Vena Cava Interruption

Surgical therapy for proximal DVT is required when patients fail anticoagulant therapy, or when there are contraindications to anticoagulant therapy. Such con-

Table 4.13 Outcome of treating patients with deep-vein thrombosis with streptokinase

		VENOGRAPHIC RESULT			
THERAPY	PATIENTS	Substantial Improvement	Partial Improvement	No Change	Progression
Streptokinase	229	47%	17%	34%	2%
Heparin	171	4%	17%	74%	5%

Venograms performed within 1 week of therapy.

Reproduced with permission from Loscalzo J, Schafer AI, eds. Thrombosis and hemorrhage. 2nd ed. Philadelphia: Lippincott Williams & Wilkins, 1998. Copyright ©1998, Lippincott Williams & Wilkins Co.

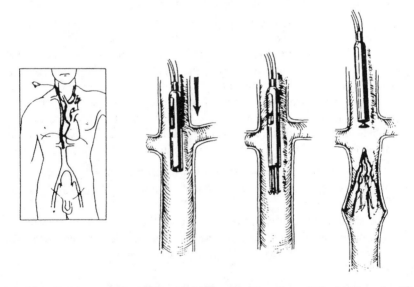

Figure 4.2. Sequence of Kimray-Greenfield filter insertion through the jugular vein. After advancing the carrier to the level of the pelvis (*left*), it is withdrawn to the third lumbar level and the stylet advanced slowly (*center*). Once the filter escapes from the carrier it springs into a self-seating position below the renal veins (*right*). (Reproduced with permission from Loscalzo J, Schafer AI, eds. Thrombosis and hemorrhage. 2nd ed. Philadelphia: Lippincott Williams & Wilkins, 1998. Copyright © 1998, Lippincott Williams & Wilkins Co.)

traindications include severe trauma (such as intracranial trauma) and a recent history of major bleeding. The procedure of choice for inferior vena cava (IVC) interruption is Kimray-Greenfield filter placement (Fig. 4.2). In the hands of an experienced person, the Kimray-Greenfield filter works very well: the IVC achieves patency in 95% of patients and there is a less than 5% risk of thromboembolism. Unfortunately, IVC flow remains decreased in almost one-half of all patients, which leads to chronic venous stasis of the legs and increased risk of recurrent DVT (28). For this reason, IVC filters are not used routinely for treating DVT.

Annotated Bibliography

1. Weinmann EE, Salzman EW. Deep-vein thrombosis. N Engl J Med 1994;331:1630–1638.

   This review paper is the gold standard, covering every clinical aspect of venous thromboembolism.

2. Morgenthaler TI, Ryu JH. Clinical characteristics of fatal pulmonary embolism in a referral hospital. Mayo Clin Proc 1995;70:417–424.

   This paper is a call to arms for physicians to develop a *high index of suspicion* for PE in hospitalized patients. Almost one-half of all patients evaluated had fatal PEs that had not even been suspected before their deaths mainly because the symptoms were often absent (only 59% had dyspnea). Most disconcerting is the observation made regarding prophylaxis: almost one-half of the patients were on adequate prophylaxis. This means that one must maintain a *high index of suspicion* even with patients receiving prophylactic therapy. It also means that one-half of at-risk inpatients are *not* being managed properly in terms of the institution of prophylactic measures.

3. Moser KM, Fedullo PF, Littlejohn JK, Crawford R. Frequent asymptomatic pulmonary embolism in patients with deep venous thrombosis. JAMA 1994;271:223–225.

   This study found that 40% of patients with DVT without any symptoms of PE had high-probability lung scan results. These results are the most recent to confirm the concept that DVT and PE are part of a single disease process—VTE.

4. Cogo A, Bernardi E, Prandoni P, et al. Acquired risk factors for deep-vein thrombosis in symptomatic outpatients. Arch Intern Med 1994;154:164–168.

   This is a retrospective and descriptive study that is important because it reminds clinicians that outpatients are also susceptible to VTE diseases when they have the risk factors that are typically evaluated within the context of sick inpatients. The risk factors most often associated with outpatients who developed DVT are immobilization, trauma, recent surgery, cancer, heart failure, lupus, and arteriopathy.

5. Hirsh J, Fuster V. Guide to anticoagulant therapy. Part 1. Heparin. Circulation 1994;89:1449–1468.

   This is an excellent review of the pathophysiology of thrombosis and the mechanism of action of heparin and heparin-like compounds. It catalogues all the thrombotic disorders (both venous and arterial) in which heparin and LMWH have been investigated. It also provides concrete recommendations for the use of heparin in different clinical settings.

6. Agnelli G, Piovella F, Buonchistiani P, et al. Enoxaparin plus compression stockings compared with compression stockings alone in the prevention of venous thromboembolism after elective neurosurgery. N Engl J Med 1998;339:80–85.

   In this multicenter study, 307 patients were randomized to placebo versus enoxaparin (40 mg, subcutaneously, daily) beginning within 24 hours of a neurosurgical procedure. All patients wore thigh-length compression stockings, and 85% of each group had follow-up bilateral venography within 10 days of the operation. Forty-two of 154 (32%) placebo-treated and 22 of 153 (17%) enoxaparin-treated patients developed DVT. Two patients in the placebo group died of PE. Four patients in the placebo group and three patients in the treatment group suffered intracranial bleeding.

7. Hull R, Raskob G, Pineo G, et al. A comparison of subcutaneous low-molecular-weight heparin with warfarin sodium for prophylaxis against deep-vein thrombosis after hip or knee implantation. N Engl J Med 1993;329:1370–1376.

   This very important paper examines the efficacy, toxicity, *and* cost-effectiveness. The results vis à vis efficacy and toxicity are unequivocal: LMWH is more efficacious (by 16%) but major bleeding developed in 2.8% of patients treated with LMWH (versus 1.2% of warfarin patients). The results regarding cost-effectiveness are inconclusive. For the bottom line, see Leclerc et al. (8).

8. Leclerc JR, Geerts WH, Desjardins L, et al. Prevention of venous thromboembolism after knee arthroplasty. A randomized, double-blind trial comparing enoxaparin with warfarin. Ann Intern Med 1996;124:619–626.

   Among 417 patients at risk, 109 of 211 warfarin recipients and 76 of 206 enoxaparin recipients developed postoperative DVT. DVT was ascertained by venography. Proximal DVT was the same in both groups (22 among warfarin-treated and 24 among enoxaparin-treated patients). Five percent of both groups had wound hematomas, and 2% of both groups had major bleeding (defined as a drop in Hgb of 2 gram % or more, or the need for at least two red cell transfusions). The conclusion was that enoxaparin is superior to warfarin (INR 2.0–3.0) at reducing all DVTs following knee arthroplasty.

9. Wells PS, Hirsh J, Anderson DR, et al. Accuracy of clinical assessment of deep-vein thrombosis. Lancet 1995;345:1326–1330.

   A clinical model to establish pre-test probability for 529 outpatients with suspected DVT was developed. Using a checklist of seven major points and five minor points (see Table 4.3), a high probability (85% with positive venogram) of having DVT was observed among patients with more than three major points, or more than two major points plus more than two minor points (and no alternative diagnosis).

10. Goldhaber SZ. Pulmonary Embolism. N Engl J Med 1998;339:93–104.

    Goldhaber, who has devoted his career to treating patients who suffer from

PE, offers a thorough review of the condition's clinical aspects, diagnostic testing, and treatment.

11. Kutinsky I, Blakley S, Roche V. Normal D-dimer levels in patients with pulmonary embolism. Arch Intern Med 1999;159:1569–1572.

    D-dimer levels were not elevated in 8 of 30 patients with angiographically confirmed PE. Therefore, the diagnosis of PE cannot be excluded by low D-dimer levels.

12. Lennox AF, Delis KT, Serunkuma S, et al. Combination of clinical risk assessment score and rapid whole blood D-dimer testing in the diagnosis of deep vein thrombosis in symptomatic patients. J Vasc Surg 1999;30:794–804.

13. Aschwanden M, Labs KH, Jeanneret C, et al. The value of rapid D-dimer testing combined with structured clinical evaluation for the diagnosis of deep vein thrombosis. J Vasc Surg 1999;30:929–935.

    Lennox et al. (12) and Aschwanden et al. (13) present data illustrating that D-dimer testing may be useful when combined with a clinical risk assessment for *excluding* the diagnosis of DVT. The results presented in these papers introduce an interesting hypothesis, but they cannot yet be taken as conclusive. The individual assessment tools are not yet reliable enough to support important life-saving clinical decisions.

14. de Valk HW, Banga JD, Wester JW, et al. Comparing subcutaneous danaparoid with intravenous unfractionated heparin for the treatment of venous thromboembolism. Ann Intern Med 1995;123:1–9.

    The heparinoid danaparoid (84% heparin sulfate, 12% dermatan sulfate, and 4% chondroitin sulfate, from the intestinal mucosa of pigs) was clearly more effective than infused unfractionated heparin when used in the induction phase of DVT and/or PE treatment (recurrence rate 13% in danaparoid group versus 28% in heparin group). Bleeding was similar in both groups. Danaparoid, like LMWH preparations, is administered by bolus injections delivered on a twice-daily schedule (intravenously initially, then subcutaneously); laboratory monitoring and dose readjustment are not required.

15. Weitz, JI. Low molecular weight heparins. N Engl J Med 1997;337:688–698.

    An excellent review that catalogues LMWH preparations and the clinical studies upon which FDA approvals and pending approvals of the drugs are based.

16. The Columbus Investigators. Low-molecular-weight heparin in the treatment of patients with venous thromboembolism. N Engl J Med 1997;337:657–669.

    These three papers (16–18) track the course of investigations that will some day lead to LMWHs replacing unfractionated heparin. In the first paper from outside the United States, an LMWH preparation not currently available in the United States (reviparin) was used to treat acute VTE. Its dosing can be standardized to all LMWH preparations: 6300 anti-factor Xa units, subcutaneously twice a day (for patients weighing more than 60 kg); 4200 units subcutaneously twice a day (weight 46 to 60 kg); 3500 units subcutaneously twice a day (35 to 45 kg). These doses are easily calculated for dalteparin and ardeparin. Enoxaparin dosing can be converted using the formula that 1000 anti-Xa units = 1 mg enoxaparin. LMWH was compared to standard heparin among 1021 randomized patients. All patients started standard warfarin within 1 to 2 days of beginning heparin. Heparin was continued for at least 5 days until the INR reached 2.0 for 2 consecutive days, and warfarin was continued for 4 months. DVT recurrence was about 5% in each group; 3.1% of the LMWH group and 2.3% of the unfractionated heparin group had major bleeding. Mortality was about 7% in each group. The conclusion is that LMWH is comparable to unfractionated heparin for the treatment of acute VTE.

17. Koopman MMW, Buller HR. Low-molecular-weight heparins in the treatment of venous thromboembolism. Ann Intern Med 1998;128:1037–1039.

An editorial by investigators outside the United States that reviews the risks-benefits of unfractionated heparin versus LMWH from many studies (including the Columbus Study). It suggests that we in the United States consider using LMWH for acute VTE because its therapeutic index is superior.

18. Gould MK, Dembitzer AD, Sanders GD, Garber AM. Low-molecular-weight heparins compared with unfractionated heparin for treatment of acute deep venous thrombosis. A cost-effectiveness analysis. Ann Intern Med 1999;130:789–809.

This paper builds on the theme that LMWH can be used for VTE, offering a theoretical cost analysis. Inpatient treatment of VTE with either LMWH or unfractionated heparin costs about the same (about $26,000). Outpatient treatment with LMWH is substantially cheaper.

19. Levine M, Gent M, Hirsh J, et al. A comparison of low-molecular-weight heparin administered primarily at home with unfractionated heparin administered in the hospital for proximal deep-vein thrombosis. N Engl J Med 1996;334:677–681.

Five hundred patients were randomly assigned to enoxaparin (1 mg/kg, subcutaneously, twice a day) or intravenous standard heparin with warfarin starting on the second day (10 mg initial dose with daily monitoring to achieve an INR of 2.0–3.0). The study drugs were discontinued when the target INR was achieved on 2 successive days. Among the 247 in the "outpatient" group, 120 were never hospitalized; the remainder had the LMWH started while they were in the hospital. There was no difference in the recurrence rate between the two groups (13 of 247 LMWH versus 17 of 253 standard heparin) or in the rate of major bleeding (5 of 247 versus 3 of 253). Thus, outpatient treatment of DVT appears to be feasible in settings where home INR monitoring systems are organized.

20. Koopman MMW, Prandoni P, Piovella F, et al. Treatment of venous thrombosis with intravenous unfractionated heparin administered in the hospital as compared with subcutaneous low-molecular-weight heparin administered at home. The Tasman Study Group. N Engl J Med 1996;334:682–687.

The results of this study support those of Levine et al. (19), and demonstrate that the home treatment program improves quality of life. It should not be long before cost-effectiveness analyses are completed and outpatient treatment of DVT becomes routine for many patients in many communities.

21. Schulman S, Rhedin A-S, Lindmarker P, Carlsson A, et al. A comparison of six weeks with six months of oral anticoagulant therapy after a first episode of venous thromboembolism. N Engl J Med 1995;332:1661–1665.

Recurrent venous thromboembolism over 2 years of follow-up was almost twice as frequent in patients treated with 6 weeks versus 6 months of warfarin (target INR of 2.0–3.0): 18.1% versus 9.5%, respectively. The data also indicated that the greatest risk for recurrence was constant for the first 6 months, suggesting that 6 months of warfarin as maintenance therapy for DVT may be better than 3 months of therapy.

22. Kearon C, Gent M, Hirsh J, et al. A comparison of three months of anticoagulation with extended anticoagulation for a first episode of idiopathic venous thromboembolism. N Engl J Med 1999;340:901–907.

In this study, 162 patients were randomly assigned to warfarin for 3 months followed by placebo for 21 months versus warfarin for 24 months. Target INR was 2.0–3.0. The study was stopped after an interim analysis, after an average of 10 months of treatment revealed that VTE recurrence was 27.4% per patient-year in placebo group and 1.3% in treatment group.

23. Prandoni P, Lensing AWA, et al. The long-term clinical course of acute deep venous thrombosis. Ann Intern Med 1996;125:1–7.

To determine the rate of recurrent DVT, post-thrombotic ("post-phlebitic") syndrome, and death, this study evaluated 355 consecutive patients over 8 years following their first episode of symptomatic DVT. The cumulative incidence of recurrence was 17.5% at 2 years, 24.6% at 5 years, and 30.3% at 8 years. Cancer and impaired coagulation inhibition were associated with increased recurrence; surgery, recent trauma, or fracture was associated with a decreased risk of recurrence. The post-thrombotic syndrome developed in 22.8% at 2 years, 28% at 5 years, and 29.1% at 8 years; it was associated with an increased risk of ipsilateral recurrence. Mortality from all causes was 30% at 8 years, with 52 of 355 dying of cancer during the 8-year follow-up period. One conclusion drawn from these data is that long-term anticoagulation may be beneficial in patients with cancer who have suffered from their first DVT. This remains to be proven, however.

24. Hirsh J, Hoak J. AHA medical/scientific statement: management of deep venous thrombosis and pulmonary embolism, a statement for health care professionals. Circulation 1996;63:2212–2245.

This is a comprehensive practical "guidebook" to the prophylaxis, diagnosis, and treatment of DVT. It presents two uniquely excellent discussions: one on the approach to alleged DVT recurrence and the other on thromboneurosis. Both of these discussions should be consulted before embarking on a complex workup or before labeling a patient as "hypercoagulable."

25. Bergqvist D, Jendteg S, Johansen L, et al. Cost of long-term complications of deep venous thrombosis of the lower extremities: an analysis of a defined population in Sweden. Ann Intern Med 1997;126:454–457.

    This is a case-control study of 257 patients with DVT. After 15 years of follow-up evaluations, 35 patients were still alive (versus 57% of the control patients). Among the DVT group members 242 complications were reported (versus 25 for the control group). The cost of managing the complications for each DVT patient during this long follow-up period was estimated as $4659 (versus $375 for control patients).

26. Brandjes DP, Büller HR, Heijboer H, et al. Randomised trial of effect of compression stockings in patients with symptomatic proximal-vein thrombosis. Lancet 1997;349:759–762.

    This study randomly assigned 194 patients with first episode DVT to wearing compression stockings during the day for 2 to 3 weeks after the acute DVT. Mild to moderate post-phlebitic syndrome was seen in 20% of the treated patients and 47% of untreated patients; a severe syndrome was seen in 11% of the treated patients versus 23% of the untreated.

27. Schulman S, Granqvist S, Holmstrom M, et al. Duration of Anticoagulation Trial Study Group. The duration of oral anticoagulant therapy after a second episode of venous thromboembolism. N Engl J Med 1997;336:393–402.

    Six months of warfarin versus indefinite anticoagulation were compared in 227 patients with a second VTE. The target INR was 2.0–2.85. In the 6-month treatment group 23 of 111 (20.7%), and in the indefinite group 3 of 116 (2.6%), had another episode of VTE over the 4-year follow-up period. Major hemorrhages developed in three patients (2.7%) in the 6-month treatment group and in 10 (8.6%) of the indefinite group. There was no difference in mortality between the two groups.

28. Decousus H, Leizorovicz A, Parent F, et al. A clinical trial of vena caval filters in the prevention of pulmonary embolism in patients with proximal deep vein thrombosis. N Engl J Med 1998;338:409–415.

    This is a complicated (and to me, befuddling) study on the use of vena caval filters plus heparin to treat acute DVT. Patients were assessed at day 12 and at 2 years. Among the 200 patients who received filters, two developed PE. Nine of the 200 patients who did not receive an IVC filter had a PE. At 2 years, 37 of the 200 filter patients versus 21 of the 200 no-filter patients had a recurrent DVT.

5

Anticoagulant Therapy

Standard treatment for venous thromboembolism is heparin followed by warfarin (see Chapter 4). To understand these antithrombotic agents and establish a background sufficient for intelligent anticipation of newer agents, a brief digression into the chemistry of heparin and warfarin follows.

Heparin

Heparin is a complex carbohydrate used to inhibit coagulation reactions. It is a natural product derived from porcine intestinal mucosa and bovine lung. Humans synthesize heparin in mast cells, but this heparin is not released in any measurable quantities, and endogenous plasma heparin levels are zero, indicating that there is no physiological role of blood heparin. An even more complex structure similar to heparin termed *heparan sulfate proteoglycan* is found in the vessel wall and may play a role in localizing the natural anticoagulant activity of antithrombin III (ATIII) to sites of disrupted vasculature (see Chapter 1). The major pharmacological effect of administered heparin is through its inhibition of the activities of thrombin and activated factors XII, XI, X, and IX. How does this work?

Figure 5.1 shows the critical pentasaccharide sequence required for the function of heparin, which is a mixture of heterogeneous polymers showing a size distribution from 4,000 to 30,000 daltons. Smaller polymers composed of oligosaccharides of less than 18 residues inhibit only factor Xa (this is the structural basis for "low-molecular-weight heparin"), whereas larger polymers with oligosaccharides greater than 18 residues inhibit factor Xa, as well as thrombin and factors XIIa, XIa, and IXa ("unfractionated heparin") (1). The obvious characteristics of the structure shown in Figure 5.1 that relate to function are the sulfate (SO_3^-) groups, which bind electrostatically (and therefore reversibly) to positively charged lysine (and arginine) groups on ATIII (Fig. 5.2). ATIII is a 58,000-dalton bean-shaped protein that binds with a 1:1 stoichiometry to thrombin and activated factors XII, XI, X, and IX. The binding of heparin to ATIII results in a conformational change in ATIII that causes the ATIII to

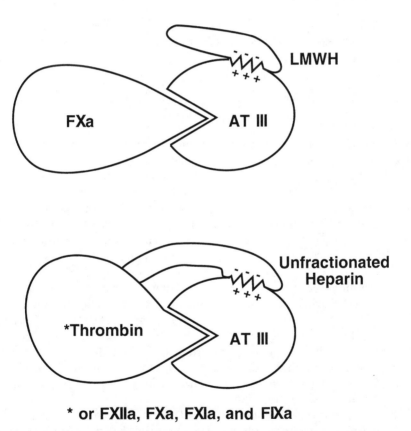

Figure 5.1. Critical pentasaccharide sequence of heparin necessary to accelerate antithrombin III activity. X—H or SO_3^-; Y—SO_3^- or $COCH_3$. (Reproduced with permission from Loscalzo J, Schafer AI, eds. Thrombosis and hemorrhage. 2nd ed. Philadelphia: Lippincott Williams & Wilkins, 1998. Copyright ©1998, Lippincott Williams & Wilkins Co.)

* or FXIIa, FXa, FXIa, and FIXa

Figure 5.2. Low-molecular-weight heparin (LMWH) binds only to antithrombin III (ATIII), triggering a conformation change in ATIII that permits it to bind only to factor Xa. Unfractionated heparin also does this, but in addition, it directly binds to both ATIII and coagulation factors XIIa, XIa, and IXa, thereby bringing enzyme (ATIII) and substrate (factors XIIa, XIa, and IXa) into juxtaposition. Therefore, unfractionated heparin inactivates thrombin and factors Xa, XIIa, XIa, and IXa. LMWH inactivates only factor Xa.

Table 5.1   Recommendations for the use of unfractionated heparin

CONDITION	EFFECTIVE HEPARIN REGIMEN
Venous thromboembolism	
Prophylaxis	5000 U subcutaneously, two or three times per day (see Chapter 4)
Treatment	Intravenous bolus 5000 U followed by 30,000–35,000 U/day intravenous infusion or 35,000–40,000 U/day by subcutaneous injection three times daily (aim for aPTT 1.5–2.5 times control)
Coronary artery disease	
Unstable angina	Intravenous bolus 5000 U followed by 32,000 U/day intravenous infusion (aim for aPTT 1.5–2.5 times control)
Acute myocardial infarction (prevent mural thrombus, reinfarction, and death)	Intravenous bolus 5000 U followed by 32,000 U/day intravenous infusion (aim for aPTT 1.5–2.5 times control)
Post-angioplasty +/- stenting (prevent restenosis and may improve mortality)	Intravenous bolus 5000 U followed by 24,000 U/day intravenous infusion (to maintain aPTT 1.5 times control)

become an active enzyme, thereby catalyzing the proteolysis and inactivation of the coagulation protein to which it is bound.

The biological behavior of heparins of different size probably relates to domain structures. Low-molecular-weight heparin has a single domain containing the pentasaccharide structure shown in Figure 5.1 that permits its interaction with ATIII complexed to factor Xa. Larger oligosaccharides (16 residues and greater) contain this domain, as well as two additional domains that permit binding to ATIII complexed to thrombin and factors XIIa, XIa, Xa, and IXa. It appears that these additional domains interact directly with the coagulation protein, forming a complex in which the pentasaccharide domain is reversibly bound to ATIII, while the two other domains bind reversibly to the coagulation protein (see Fig. 5.2). Thus, "low-molecular-weight heparin," which is composed of a heterogeneous mixture of heparin polymers with an average size of 4000 to 7000 daltons, is simply a product of depolymerization of "unfractionated heparin" by chemical or enzymatic means. This product is enriched in the domain that binds only to ATIII and is deficient in the domains that bind directly to the substrates of ATIII.

The indications for using standard unfractionated heparin are listed in Table 5.1. Problems associated with standard heparin therapy are common and include particularly

1. unpredictable levels of anticoagulation reflected in unpredictable aPTT response

2. close laboratory monitoring required

3. bleeding

4. thrombocytopenia

5. osteoporosis

Unpredictable blood heparin levels leading to unpredictable swings in the aPTT when one is trying to rapidly achieve and then maintain a therapeutic aPTT (1.5 to 2.5 times control) can be a frustrating and dangerous situation. The reason for this is that heparin binds to many plasma proteins and the vascular endothelium, and every lot of heparin is different in this regard, resulting in altered bioavailability and clearance. This leads to the need for close laboratory monitoring (which is sometimes ignored because of its monotony), and increases the likelihood of under-anticoagulation (with its attendant risk of recurrent thrombosis) and over-anticoagulation (with its attendant risk of hemorrhage). Patients who develop a major hemorrhage (variously defined, but generally involving at least a decrease in blood hemoglobin of 2 g/dL) while on heparin must have the heparin stopped and its activity reversed. Heparin activity is reversed by protamine, which is heavily positively charged and binds to the negatively charged domains (including the pentasaccharide domains) on heparin. Protamine is used at a dose of 1 mg per 100 U of circulating heparin, and it should be administered by infusion over 10 to 20 minutes in order to avoid hypotension.

Heparin-associated thrombocytopenia results from heparin binding to platelets, forming a hapten that stimulates an antibody response. Small decreases in platelet counts are common among patients receiving standard heparin. The importance of these decreases and their relationship to the potentially dangerous syndrome of *heparin-induced thrombocytopenia with thrombosis* (HITT) will be discussed in Chapter 14. Heparin-induced osteoporosis can be avoided by keeping full-dose heparin treatment under 14 days. For adjusted-dose subcutaneous heparin (i.e., used as maintenance treatment for venous thrombosis), doses of 20,000 U/24 hours for 3 months or less appear to not cause osteoporosis.

Low-Molecular-Weight Heparin

Low-molecular-weight heparin (LMWH) appears to offer advantages regarding each of the problems associated with heparin therapy except osteoporosis. LMWH has less binding to plasma proteins and vascular endothelium, resulting in more predictable bioavailability and pharmacokinetic properties. It requires *no* laboratory monitoring. For comparably efficacious responses, LMWH produces fewer hemorrhagic sequelae; during initial therapy for proximal vein thrombosis, 1 of 213 patients receiving LMWH had major bleeding, compared with 11 of 219 patients receiving standard infused heparin (2). Heparin-induced thrombocytopenia developed in 9 of 332 patients receiving standard heparin versus none of 333 patients receiving LMWH (3). The effect of chronic administration of LMWH on bone integrity is uncertain; until studies disprove it, we must assume that long-term LMWH causes osteoporosis.

Table 5.2   Low-molecular-weight heparins and heparinoids

AGENT	BRAND NAME	SIZE	INDICATION	DOSE	COST
Enoxaparin	Lovenox	4000 daltons	Prevent DVT after hip replacement or knee replacement	30 mg sc q 12 h	~$30/day
			Prevent DVT after abdominal surgery	40 mg sc q 24 h	~$20/day
			Treat DVT in outpatients	1 mg/kg q 12 h	~$80/day
			Treatment of DVT without or with PE in hospitalized patients	1 mg/kg q 12 h or 1.5 mg/kg q 24 h	~$80/day ~$60/day
Dalteparin	Fragmin	5000 daltons	Prevent DVT after abdominal surgery	2500–5000 anti-Xa U sc q 24 h	~$12/day
Ardeparin	Normiflo	6000 daltons	Prevent DVT after knee replacement	50 anti-Xa U/kg sc q 12 h	~$30/day
Tinzaparin	Innohep	5000 daltons	Treatment of DVT without or with PE	175 anti-Xa U/kg sc q 24 h	~$100/day
Danaparoid	Orgaran	5500 daltons	Prevent DVT after hip replacement	750 anti-Xa U bid	~$200/day

Although there are at least 11 LMWH preparations available worldwide, only four are currently available in the United States (Table 5.2). Enoxaparin (Lovenox; Rhône-Poulec Rorer) is approved for use to prevent deep venous thrombosis (DVT) after hip or knee replacement or after abdominal surgery beginning within 24 hours of the operation, and to treat DVT in both inpatients and outpatients. Dalteparin (Fragmin; Pharmacia/Upjohn) is approved for use to prevent DVT among patients undergoing abdominal surgery; it is administered as a single 2500 IU (anti-factor Xa) subcutaneous injection for 7 to 10 days after surgery. Ardeparin (Normiflo; Wyeth-Ayerst) is approved for use to prevent DVT in patients undergoing knee replacement; it is begun post-operatively at a dose of 50 anti-Xa IU/kg subcutaneously every 12 hours and continued for 7 to 10 days. Tinzaparin (Innohep; Dupont) is approved for the treatment of DVT without or with PE; it is administered as a single daily dose of 175 anti-Xa units/kg for at least 6 days and until the patient is adequately anticoagulated with warfarin.

In general, LMWHs appear to be a reasonable substitute for all indicated uses of unfractionated heparin. They have been approved for use by the U.S. Food and Drug Administration mainly in the prophylaxis setting, although tinzaparin and enoxaparin have recently been approved for use in patients with DVT or pulmonary embolism (PE). It is likely that LMWH will replace standard heparin in all of its indications. The doses of the LMWH used in the treatment of venous thromboembolism, atrial fibrillation, or acute coronary artery syndromes are greater than doses used for prophylaxis.

Heparinoids

The recent elucidation of the structural aspects of heparin responsible for its anticoagulant properties has formed the basis for a new group of anticoagulant drugs undergoing large-scale clinical investigation. To understand the biological basis of these "heparinoids," we must first introduce a new character in the cast of molecules involved in the ongoing saga of heparin: *heparin cofactor II*. This is a molecule discovered by its capacity to bind directly to heparin. In the presence of heparin, heparin cofactor II binds to and cleaves thrombin; it has no effect on other coagulation proteins. The affinity of heparin for ATIII is much greater than its affinity for heparin cofactor II, and heparin cofactor II probably is not involved in the anticoagulant actions of standard heparin therapy.

It turns out, however, that polysaccharides other than heparin also bind to heparin cofactor II, and that this binding activates heparin cofactor II to cleave and inactivate thrombin. The polysaccharides that greatly accelerate the proteolysis of thrombin by heparin cofactor II are termed *heparinoids*. Heparinoids are a heterogeneous mixture of proteoglycans composed mainly of *glycosaminoglycans*. Within this mixture, the glycosaminoglycan most responsible for heparin cofactor II activation is *dermatan sulfate*.

The only heparinoid available in the United States is *danaparoid* (see Table 5.2). Danaparoid is composed of a mixture of sulfated glycosaminoglycans: heparan sulfate (84%), dermatan sulfate (12%) and chondroitin sulfate (4%). Danaparoid appears to be an effective anticoagulant possessing many of the advantages of LMWH (particularly standard dosing eliminating the need for aPTT monitoring) without the risk of heparin-induced thrombocytopenia, and its boundaries of indication for use are gradually expanding to include those of standard heparin. It is effective as an anticoagulant because it is composed of a small fraction (<5%) of heparan sulfate containing the pentasaccharide structure that mediates ATIII-induced factor Xa inactivation, *plus* the dermatan sulfate that mediates heparin cofactor II–induced thrombin inactivation. It is approved for use in the United States for the prevention of DVT after hip replacement surgery, where it is given at a dose of 750 anti-Xa units by subcutaneous injection, twice daily.

Warfarin

Warfarin or related chemicals (Fig. 5.3) interfere with coagulation by mimicking vitamin K and competing for an epoxide reductase required for reducing an inactive vitamin K precursor to active vitamin K (*hydroquinone*). Figure 5.4 schematizes this process and shows that the result is the inhibition of gamma carboxylation required to activate coagulation factors II, VII, IX, and X, as well as the anticoagulant proteins C and S. Gamma carboxylation is the addition of a carboxyl group to the gamma position of glutamic acid residues present in the coagulant or anticoagulant protein (Fig. 5.5). The gamma carboxyglutamyl residues (termed *Gla*) bind calcium, resulting in the proper assembly of the coagulation complex on phospholipid surfaces (see Chapter 1).

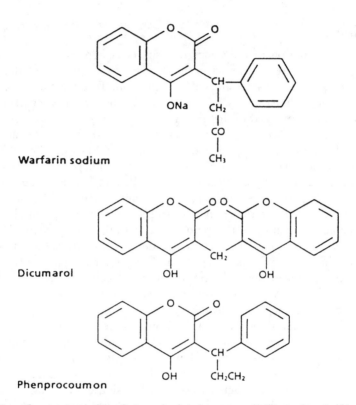

Figure 5.3. The structure of warfarin and related compounds. (Reproduced with permission from Loscalzo J, Schafer AI, eds. Thrombosis and hemorrhage. 2nd ed. Philadelphia: Lippincott Williams & Wilkins, 1998. Copyright ©1998, Lippincott Williams & Wilkins Co.)

Warfarin leads to inadequate gamma carboxylation (most coagulation factors require at least 10 Gla residues to function optimally), as well as decreased hepatic synthesis (perhaps due to degradation of inadequately carboxylated protein). The result is an increase in the prothrombin time (PT) and, eventually, the aPTT. To standardize the warfarin effect on coagulation, clinical laboratories now report an *international normalized ratio* (INR), which attempts to eradicate the influence of variable potency of thromboplastins used to trigger the PT reaction (see Chapter 2). The INR = $(PT_{PATIENT} / PT_{CONTROL})^{ISI}$ where the ISI is the *international sensitivity index* of thromboplastin used in the coagulation laboratory. Figure 5.6 graphs the relationship between the PT ratio and the INR at varying ISIs. Table 5.3 shows the current indications for warfarin therapy, and the target INR for each indication.

Any presentation of warfarin anticoagulation is accompanied by a list of medications that potentiate or inhibit its action. Table 5.4 lists some of the most common drug interactions. It is also useful to note that older patients are gen-

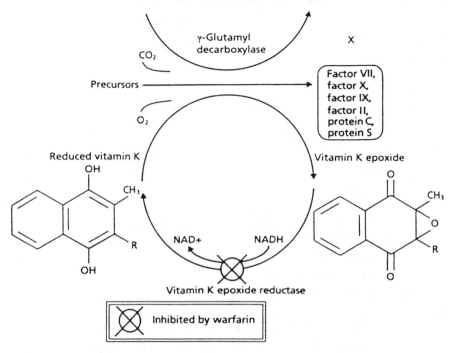

Figure 5.4. Warfarin works by blocking the vitamin K epoxide reductase and thereby preventing the generation of the active vitamin K species. (Reproduced with permission from Loscalzo J, Schafer AI, eds. Thrombosis and hemorrhage. 2nd ed. Philadelphia: Lippincott Williams & Wilkins, 1998. Copyright ©1998, Lippincott Williams & Wilkins Co.)

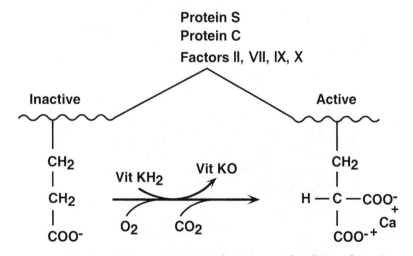

Figure 5.5. Reduced vitamin K participates in the gamma carboxylation of protein C, protein S, and coagulation factors II, VII, IX, and X. The gamma carboxylation forms a pocket for binding calcium ions on the proteins, neutralizing the acidic glutamic acid residues, and permitting the interaction of the proteins with phospholipid surfaces. The assembly of the coagulation reactions on the phospholipid surface is required for fast and efficient catalysis.

Table 5.3 Indications for warfarin anticoagulation and their target INR

CONDITION	INTERNATIONAL NORMALIZED RATIO[a]	
	Minimal Effective	Recommended
Deep-vein thrombosis		
Prevention	1.5–2.5	2.0–3.0[b]
Treatment	2.0–2.3	2.0–3.0
Atrial fibrillation: prevention of systemic embolism	1.5–2.5[c]	2.0–3.0
Cardiac valve replacement		
Tissue valves	2.0–2.3	2.0–4.5
Mechanical valves	1.9–3.6	3.0–4.5
Cerebral embolism	Not evaluated	—
Native valvular heart disease	Not evaluated	—

[a] For thromboplastin with an international sensitivity index of 2.3, the international normalized ratios (INRs) and the corresponding prothrombin time ratios are as follows:

INR	1.5	2.0	2.5	3.0	3.5	4.0	4.5	5.0
Prothrombin time ratio	1.20	1.35	1.49	1.61	1.72	1.83	1.92	2.01

[b] A lower range may be effective.
[c] Based on an international sensitivity index of 2.3.

Reproduced with permission from Loscalzo J, Schafer AI, eds. Thrombosis and hemorrhage. 2nd ed. Philadelphia: Lippincott Williams & Wilkins, 1998:1164. Copyright ©1998, Lippincott Williams & Wilkins Co.

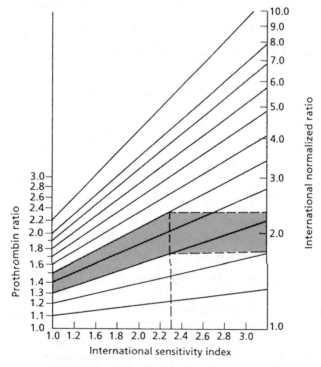

Figure 5.6.   The relationship between the prothrombin time ratio ($PT_{PATIENT}/PT_{CONTROL}$) and the international normalized ratio (INR) at varying international sensitivity indexes (ISIs). (Reproduced with permission from Loscalzo J, Schafer AI, eds. Thrombosis and hemorrhage. 2nd ed. Philadelphia: Lippincott Williams & Wilkins, 1998. Copyright ©1998, Lippincott Williams & Wilkins Co.)

Table 5.4 Some drugs that interact with warfarin

PHARMACOKINETIC (DRUGS THAT CHANGE WARFARIN LEVELS)	PHARMACODYNAMIC (DRUGS THAT DO NOT CHANGE WARFARIN LEVELS)	MECHANISM UNKNOWN (DRUGS WHOSE EFFECT ON WARFARIN IS UNKNOWN)
Prolongs prothrombin time	**Prolongs prothrombin time**	**Prolongs prothrombin time**
Stereoselective inhibition of clearance of S isomer	Inhibits cyclic interconversion of vitamin K	Evidence for interaction convincing
• Phenylbutazone	• 2nd and 3rd generation cephalosporins	• Erythromycin
• Metronidazole	Other mechanisms	• Anabolic steroids
• Sulfinpyrazone	• Clofibrate	Evidence for interaction less convincing
• Trimethoprim-sulfamethoxazole	Inhibits blood coagulation	• Ketoconazole
• Disulfiram	• Heparin	• Fluconazole
Stereoselective inhibition of clearance of R isomer	Increases metabolism of coagulation factors	• Piroxicam
• Cimetidine[a]	• Thyroxine	• Tamoxifen
• Omeprazole[a]	**Inhibits platelet function**	• Quinidine
Nonstereoselective inhibitions of clearance of	• Aspirin	• Vitamin E (megadose)
R and S isomers	• Other nonsteroidal anti-inflammatory drugs	• Phenytoin
• Amiodarone	• Ticlopidine	**Reduces prothrombin time**
Reduces prothrombin time	• Moxalactam	• Penicillins
Reduces absorption	• Carbenicillin and high doses of other penicillins	• Griseofulvin[b]
• Cholestyramine		
Increases metabolic clearance		
• Barbiturates		
• Rifampin		
• Griseofulvin		
• Carbamazepine		

[a] Causes minimal prolongation of the prothrombin time.

[b] Has been proposed to cause increased metabolic clearance.

Reproduced with permission from Loscalzo J, Schafer AI, eds. Thrombosis and hemorrhage. 2nd ed. Philadelphia: Lippincott Williams & Wilkins, 1998:1168. Copyright ©1998, Lippincott Williams & Wilkins Co.

erally more sensitive to warfarin (4). Close monitoring of the INR after beginning warfarin, maintaining the INR within the desired range, and avoiding antiplatelet agents (such as aspirin) minimize the risks of bleeding with warfarin therapy. When bleeding develops, it can be reversed immediately by giving factors II, VII, IX, and X (in fresh frozen plasma). The half-lives of these factors are: II, 72 hours; VII, 6 hours; IX, 24 hours; and X, 36 hours. Therefore, it may take at least 72 hours to overcome a warfarin effect with vitamin K injections. Standard dose vitamin K (10 mg subcutaneously each day) can render a person warfarin-resistant for 6 weeks or longer. One can perhaps avoid this, and effectively (but slowly) reverse warfarin toxicity, with the use of 10 to 100 µg of vitamin K administered daily by subcutaneous injection until the INR approaches the desired therapeutic target. When an INR exceeds 5.0 in a clinically asymptomatic patient, it can be brought back to the desired target INR by withholding one or two doses of warfarin *and* administering a single 2.5-mg oral dose of vitamin K (5).

Annotated Bibliography

1. Hirsh J, Fuster V. Guide to anticoagulant therapy part 1: heparin. Circulation 1994;89:1449–1468.

   A broad review of heparin preparations, including the LMWHs, from their biochemistry to their clinical pharmacology.

2. Hull RD, Raskob GE, Pineo GF, et al. Subcutaneous low-molecular-weight heparin compared with continuous intravenous heparin in the treatment of proximal vein thrombosis. New Engl J Med 1992;326:975–982.

   LMWH is at least as effective and safe as standard unfractionated heparin: the recurrence was 6 of 213 patients for LMWH and 15 of 219 patients for standard heparin; the major bleeding was 1 of 213 patients for LMWH and 11 of 219 patients for standard heparin.

3. Warkentin TE, Levine MN, Hirsh J, et al. Heparin-induced thrombocytopenia in patients with low-molecular-weight heparin or un-fractionated heparin. New Engl J Med 1995;332:1330–1335.

   Heparin-induced thrombocytopenia (HIT) was defined as a decrease of platelet count less than 150,000/µL beginning 5 or more days after therapy was started *plus* heparin-dependent IgG antibodies. HIT occurred in 9 of the 322 patients receiving standard heparin (8 of 9 suffered associated thrombosis) and in none of the 333 patients who received LMWH. Heparin-associated antibodies were found in 7.8% of all persons treated with unfractionated heparin and 2.2% of persons receiving LMWH.

4. Gurwitz JH, Avorn J, Ross-Degnan D, et al. Aging and the anticoagulant response to warfarin therapy. Ann Intern Med 1992;116:901–904.

   A retrospective analysis of 530 patients monitored in an anticoagulation clinic over 10 years. For a single dose of warfarin, the PT was prolonged more with each decade of life beginning at age 50. Weight and therapy duration greater than 6 months were associated with a decreased warfarin response. Older patients need their INR watched closely.

5. Weibert RT, Le DT, Kayser SR, Rapaport SI. Correction of excessive anticoagulation with low-dose oral vitamin K_1. Ann Intern Med 1997;125:959–962.

In 68 of 71 patients who had their warfarin held for one to two doses because of a supratherapeutic INR, oral vitamin K lowered the INR from 10.0 to 5.0 to less than 5.0 without causing any warfarin resistance.

6

Arterial Thrombosis

Thrombosis of the arteries remains the most common disease process afflicting adults in the United States. Thrombosis of the coronary arteries affects millions of people, with syndromes related to myocardial ischemia or infarction resulting in morbidity in over 5 million people per year. Over 500,000 people in the United States die annually from the complications of coronary artery thrombosis. In addition to these staggering figures for coronary artery disease (CAD), thrombosis in the carotid arteries and its branches results in death and disability for over 100,000 and one-half million people, respectively, annually in the United States. Last, but perhaps not least, are peripheral arterial diseases. The mortality from vaso-occlusion of the large arteries (the aorta and its proximal branches) is less than the mortality from diseases of the coronary and cerebral arteries, but overall more people probably suffer from diseases of the peripheral arteries than from both coronary and carotid diseases combined. The age-adjusted prevalence of peripheral arterial diseases in the United States is about 12%. Peripheral arterial disease (PAD) directly affects mortality (threefold increased risk of dying, independent of risk associated with CAD). It is also important to emphasize that PAD is an important "red flag" identifying previously unrecognized CAD: almost all patients with symptomatic PAD have CAD, which puts them at a dramatically increased risk of dying.

The pathophysiology of arterial thrombosis in the overwhelming majority of cases involves *atherothrombosis*, a pathogenetic process encompassing chronic progressive atherosclerosis punctuated by one of two (or both) acute processes: 1) plaque rupture and 2) platelet thrombus formation in areas of progressive stenosis.

Platelet thrombus formation is the predominant final common pathway for arterial thrombosis, whatever the antecedent event (see Chapter 1), including thrombosis initiated by atherosclerotic plaque rupture. Therefore, most therapeutic strategies for treating and preventing arterial thrombosis are directed at limiting (or eradicating) platelet-dependent thrombus formation. An arterial thrombus is, however, a dynamic process; as luminal narrowing progresses, so does the importance of the soluble coagulation system. Fibrin production is almost always a critical, albeit late, component of arterial thromboses. Directing treatments at either minimizing fibrin accrual (e.g., heparin) or removing deposited fibrin (e.g., thrombolytics) are therefore reasonable and established therapeutic strategies. They are not, however, nearly effective enough (too little, too late), and one must consider prophylactic measures as the major attack point against arterial thrombosis.

Risk Factors: The Primary Prevention of Atherosclerosis

Most risk factors for atherosclerosis are highly publicized and well-known by physicians and non-physicians alike. Some are clearly established—smoking, diabetes, hyperlipidemia (including high levels of serum total cholesterol, low density lipoprotein, triglycerides, apolipoprotein B and lipoprotein(a)), low levels of serum high density lipoprotein, hypertension, aging, family history, physical inactivity, and gender. Others are less clearly established—obesity, coagulation factor levels, and hyperhomocystinemia.

Cataloguing risk factors is of no use to the clinician unless knowledge of a risk factor contributes to patient management. How can risk factor assessment help an individual patient? First (and the first learned by medical students), it helps us to develop a diagnostic and/or therapeutic plan for patients who have a history suggesting ischemia of the heart, brain, viscera, or limbs. An elderly man who presents with atypical chest pain is more likely to have CAD if he gives a history including several risk factors. Is this sufficient information to establish a diagnosis? Of course not! But, if the diagnostic testing demonstrates CAD, one can next attempt to affect outcome by modifying risk factors.

When a risk factor is altered prior to any established disease this is called *primary prevention*. When it is altered after a disease process has struck, it is called *secondary prevention*. Various risk factors, including those that permit intervention, are listed in Table 6.1. Please note that the possibility of intervention does not guarantee a high probability of effective intervention, and in every case an intervention is *easier said than done*, generally requiring a solid health care support system and a highly motivated patient.

Atherosclerotic Arterial Thrombosis

Clinical syndromes related to atherosclerotic diseases of the coronary, cerebral, and peripheral arteries tend to be grouped based on whether the vaso-occlusion leads to ischemia or infarction. In every case, however, similar pathogenetic factors are involved, and the difference between ischemia (e.g., *stable angina*, a *transient ischemic attack*, or *claudication*) and infarction (e.g., *myocardial infarction*, *stroke*, or *limb infarction*) is probably due to the magnitude and duration of the atherothrombotic processes associated with the acute event.

If one looks back at the pathogenesis of acute arterial vaso-occlusion from the vantage point of successful interventions, one can identify trigger phenomena and rank the relative significance of the various coagulation pathways described in Chapter 1. Figuring out triggers and resulting factors that main-

Table 6.1   Some cardiovascular risk factors and the relative success (compliance and/or effectiveness) of standard interventions used for these risk factors

ATHEROSCLEROSIS RISK FACTOR	INTERVENTION	RELATIVE SUCCESS
Family history	None	—
Age	None	—
Lipoprotein (a)	Estrogen (?)	–/+
Postmenopausal	Estrogen replacement	–/+
Male central obesity	Weight loss	+
Diabetes mellitus	Tight control of glucose levels	+
Sedentary life style	Exercise	+
Total serum cholesterol/high LDL	Diet and/or medications	++
Smoking	Quitting	++
Low HDL cholesterol	Medications	++
Hypertriglyceridemia	Diet and/or medications	++
Hypertension	Antihypertensive medications	+++
Hyperhomocystinemia	Folic acid, vitamin B_{12}, and pyridoxine	+++

Abbreviations: HDL = high-density lipoprotein; LDL = low-density lipoprotein.

tain or amplify the triggering event is absolutely critical to devising rational therapeutic interventions.

The Triggering Event and Primary Prevention

The triggering event is platelet adhesion, release, and activation (see Fig. 1.2) developing in the setting of progressive arterial stenosis and plaque rupture. The mechanisms by which these three responses develop are fairly well understood, and this understanding forms the basis for current and future therapeutic interventions with *antiplatelet agents* (see Chapter 7). Figure 7.1 schematizes the chain reactions leading to platelet thrombus formation and identifies points of therapeutic intervention. Currently, primary prevention with aspirin (ASA) is established for decreasing the risk of myocardial infarction among adult women and men, and for decreasing the risk of stroke in women and men who have experienced transient ischemic attacks (1). Other medical interventions, as well as other potential indications for ASA in primary prevention of cerebrovascular and peripheral vascular disease, are under investigation. There is no evidence for other anticoagulant therapy offering primary protection against acute arterial syndromes leading to ischemia of the heart, brain, viscera, or limbs.

Acute Arterial Ischemia and Infarction: Antithrombotic Interventions

Platelets trigger an acute arterial thrombosis. As vaso-occlusion progresses, rheological factors associated with decreased flow permit the assembly of the soluble coagulation apparatus on the platelet thrombus and adjacent damaged vessel wall. This leads to the formation of insoluble fibrin deposited within the vessel lumen, further compromising flow and placing the patient at risk for end-organ infarction. This pathogenetic scheme applies to large arteries of the heart, brain, viscera, and limbs, and it is therefore reasonable to consider that treatment approaches are the same for CAD, cerebrovascular diseases, and PAD. To some degree this is true, but subtle differences often exist in the components of Virchow's triad in different tissues. These differences can lead to different responses to a therapeutic intervention. It therefore is advisable to scrutinize the literature for assessing the therapeutic index of every intervention that you are considering for your patient.

One important example of differing results using a single intervention in differing arterial beds is the effect of thrombolytic therapy on arterial thrombosis of the coronary and cerebral vessels. The MAST-I (Multicentre Acute Stroke Trial, Italy) study, which randomized 622 patients to placebo, ASA, streptokinase (SK), or ASA + SK, showed that 1,500,000 units of intravenous SK administered within 6 hours of the onset of a focal neurological deficit, when it was given with 300 mg ASA daily, worsened mortality at 10 days (54/156 versus 20/156 in untreated group), even though there was an overall small improvement in mortality at 60 days (99 of 156 dead in SK + ASA group versus 106 of 156 in the untreated group) (2). In contrast, numerous studies show that intravenous streptokinase improves short-term and long-term survival in patients with acute myocardial infarction (MI). For example, ISIS-2 (Second International Study of Infarct Survival) showed that 1,500,000 units of SK, administered intravenously a median of 5 hours after the onset of symptoms, decreased 35-day mortality from 13.2% to 10.4% among 8600 patients with acute MI randomly assigned to placebo or SK; also, ASA (160 mg per day) + SK decreased mortality further to 8.0% among the 4292 patients who received the combination (3). These differing results using an almost identical intervention probably reflect that blood flow to the brain is extremely brisk (consuming about 20% of the cardiac output), and that stroke damages cerebral microvascular blood vessels, which leads to a greater risk of intracerebral hemorrhage when pharmacologic fibrinolysis is employed. Of note is that thrombolytics administered for coronary artery thrombosis also lead to intracerebral hemorrhage (<1% of patients who get SK), but this risk is clearly outweighed by the benefits of restoring coronary artery blood flow.

Coronary Artery Thrombosis

Clinical Presentation

The most obvious clinical manifestation of coronary artery thrombosis is chest pain. Myocardial ischemia can also lead to dysfunction of a heart chamber or to an arrhythmia, including sudden death from ventricular fibrillation. The duration of chest pain often reflects the magnitude of the thrombosis and is inversely related to the reversibility of the damage to the myocardium: the longer the ischemia, the greater the likelihood of infarction and permanent myocardial dysfunction even when an acute thrombus is eliminated.

Diagnostic Studies

The diagnosis of acute myocardial infarction (MI) is based on symptoms, signs, electrocardiogram (ECG) results, and elevated heart creatine kinase isoenzyme (CPK-MB) and/or troponin levels. Once MI has been established, one must next contemplate the extent and magnitude of the patient's coronary artery disease.

Noninvasive testing with an exercise tolerance test (ETT) or a thallium ETT provides diagnostic and prognostic information. This information is also provided by left heart catheterization with coronary angiography and ventriculography. Coronary angiography not only provides diagnostic and prognostic information, but also can set up an angioplasty and/or stenting procedure when one is indicated. Up to 50% of all diagnostic heart catheterizations result in a therapeutic procedure.

For routine angiography, 2000–5000 U of unfractionated heparin is infused. If the catheterization procedure is expected to last less than 20 minutes, it is sometimes done without anticoagulation. When balloon dilatation and/or stenting is performed, patients routinely receive 10,000–15,000 U of intravenous heparin titrated to an activated clotting time (ACT) of more than 300 seconds. The major complication of heparin given to support cardiac catheterization is bleeding at the site of the arterial puncture (usually femoral). Note that heparin-associated thrombocytopenia can occur after short intravenous infusions (or even a single subcutaneous injection) of heparin (see Chapter 14).

There are many noninvasive diagnostic studies to establish the presence and severity of CAD. (A discussion of the methods employed and predictive value of each diagnostic test is beyond the scope of this text.) Remember that the predictive value of a test depends on the a priori probability of the disease being present, so an exercise ECG, although it is less sensitive than a nuclear isotope study, may be extremely predictive in an at-risk patient with a normal resting ECG and classic angina (in whom there is a high pre-test probability of having CAD). *Bayes's theorem* teaches us that the more sensitive a test, the more predictive a positive test will be among patients with an atypical presentation (such as atypical chest pain) (Table 6.2). But, alas, increased test sensitivity is always accompanied by decreased test specificity, so beware of the false-positive result.

In general, there are two types of tests: myocardial perfusion studies (e.g., thallium or technetium-99) and ventricular wall motion studies (e.g., two-dimensional echocardiography). These studies are performed on patients capable or incapable of exercise. Among patients who can exercise, a treadmill is used to increase myocardial work. Among patients who cannot exercise, intravenous dipyridamole or adenosine is used with nuclear studies, and intra-

Table 6.2 **Bayes's theorem of post-test probability**
(Or, what is the predictive value of the test I'm ordering?)

Background equations

Sensitivity = True positive/True positive + False negatives

Specificity = True negative/True negative + False positive

Positive predictive value = True positive/True positive + False positive

Negative predictive value = True negative/True negative + False negative

Bayesian equations

Probability of disease with a positive test =

(Sensitivity)(Prevalence)/(Sensitivity)(Prevalence) + (1 − Specificity)(1 − Prevalence)

Probability of no disease with a negative test =

(1 − Sensitivity)(Prevalence)/(1 − Sensitivity)(Prevalence) + (Specificity)(1 − Prevalence)

venous dobutamine is used with echocardiography. These agents are administered to increase coronary artery flow, and thereby unmask significant coronary artery stenosis. Remember that the diagnostic value of these noninvasive studies is measured relative to the information derived from coronary angiography, which remains the gold standard despite great technological progress in noninvasive cardiology.

Antithrombotic Therapies

Primary Prevention

ASPIRIN 325 mg orally every other day

The Physicians Health Study (PHS) evaluated 22,701 healthy male physicians (4). These men were evaluated over an average of 5 years, and they took either placebo or 325 mg of ASA every other day. The risk of MI was significantly reduced by 44% in the ASA group, apparent only among those who were 50 years of age and older. There was no effect on overall mortality. There was a small statistically insignificant increase in the risk of hemorrhagic stroke and ulcer among the ASA users.

Other studies support the conclusions of the PHS and extend their findings to all men and women, including those without clinically apparent ischemic heart disease. The greatest benefit, however, may be derived by males 50 years and older who have risk factors for CAD. The optimal dose of ASA in this setting has not been established, but it appears to be less than 325 mg per day. I recommend 325 mg every other day or 81 mg every day. ASA should probably not be given to people with active (or historic) gastrointestinal bleeding or thrombocytopenia; or a history of hemorrhagic stroke or a bleeding disorder; or to those receiving warfarin.

Stable Angina Pectoris

ASPIRIN 325 mg orally every other day

The Physicians' Health Study demonstrated that ASA, 325 mg every other day, reduced the risk of first MI by 87% among male physicians with chronic stable angina (5).

Unstable Angina

ASPIRIN 160 mg orally day 1, followed by 81 mg every day

ENOXAPARIN 1 mg/kg subcutaneous every 12 hours

After 4 to 6 days of pharmacologic treatment for unstable angina, patients should be divided into two groups based on risk. Low-risk patients are those without rest angina who rapidly stabilize on this treatment; they are managed chronically with ASA. High-risk patients are those with rest angina whose chest pain is more difficult to manage medically. These patients often benefit from coronary angiography leading to bypass grafting, angioplasty, or stenting. If these therapies are not advisable, high-risk patients may benefit from long-term ASA therapy plus warfarin for at least 3 months (aiming for an INR of 2.0–3.0) (6).

Combined ASA plus heparin appears to be the best intervention to minimize the risk for MI in patients with unstable angina (7). Note that abrupt discontinuation of heparin may result in a dangerous reactivation of ischemia, and that ASA prevents this (7). The doses of ASA that have been shown to be effective in this setting range from 75 to 1300 mg/day. Smaller doses are theoretically superior because they show an improved therapeutic index, in part because smaller doses permanently inhibit platelet cyclooxygenase activity (thereby inhibiting the production of proaggregatory and vasoconstricting thromboxane A_2) while only temporarily inhibiting vascular endothelial cyclooxygenase (thereby allowing relatively preserved prostacyclin synthesis, which is antiaggregatory and vasodilating). There are few, if any, absolute contraindications to initiating these medications. The therapeutic index of antithrombotic therapy for unstable angina is decreased in patients with active gastrointestinal bleeding and recent brain trauma or hemorrhage; these patients probably should not receive ASA plus heparin.

Can we do better? Maybe—but a conclusive answer is currently unavailable. There are more potent platelet antagonists, such as the glycoprotein (GP) IIb-IIIa receptor blockers, which interfere with the final common pathway of platelet aggregation (see Fig. 7.1). At least three compounds have demonstrated efficacy in this setting and have improved mortality rates (8). Two of these agents, tirofiban (Aggrastat, Merck) and eptifibatide (Cor Therapeutics) have recently been approved by the U.S. Food and Drug Administration for use in this setting, and it is reasonable to add one of these agents to enoxaparin and aspirin when the clinical syndrome is recalcitrant.

What about other heparins or new anticoagulants? Recent reports indicate that enoxaparin, a low-molecular-weight heparin (LMWH), is superior to standard unfractionated heparin for patients with unstable angina; the LMWH dalteparin is also better than unfractionated heparin but perhaps not as good as enoxaparin (9,10). Recombinant hirudin, a leech anticoagulant protein that inhibits thrombin's effect on fibrinogen and platelets, appears to have efficacy comparable to heparin (11), but results with hirudin as well as other direct thrombin inhibitors fail to show that these new agents have a therapeutic index clearly superior to heparins (12).

Acute MI

> ASPIRIN > 160 mg orally every day (chewable is preferred for first dose)
>
> + HEPARIN (5000 U bolus followed by 1300 U/hour; aPTT 2.5 × control)

This program is recommended for *all patients with MI, whether or not they receive thrombolytics.* In the Second International Study of Infarct Survival (ISIS-2), 160 mg per day of enteric-coated ASA reduced mortality from 11.8% to 9.4% (13). Heparin should be used in all patients with a large transmural (Q wave) anterior wall MI because it prevents the development of mural thrombi in patients with anterior wall MI. Studies before the era of fibrinolytic therapy suggest that heparin generally improves survival, so heparin is recommended for all MI patients not receiving thrombolytics or undergoing angioplasty. Tirofiban or eptifibatide has been shown to prevent acute ischemic events in non-Q-wave infarction and in unstable angina, and in some institutions these agents are used routinely in such patients. Platelet GP IIb-IIIa antagonists should not be used with thrombolytic therapy. Heparin should probably be continued until the patient has stabilized, and ASA should probably be continued throughout the patient's life.

There are no definitive data that long-term anticoagulation with warfarin is beneficial for patients who have survived the MI. It has been recommended, however, that 3 months of warfarin therapy, aiming for an INR of 2.0–3.0, should be considered for patients with anterior wall Q-wave MI. This will be discussed further under "Secondary Prevention". There are no published studies demonstrating the superiority of any new antithrombotics in this setting.

Acute MI with Thrombolysis

> tPA 15 mg intravenous bolus, followed by 0.75 mg/kg (not to exceed 50 mg) intravenous infusion over 30 minutes, followed by 0.50 mg/kg (not to exceed 35 mg) intravenous infusion over the next 60 minutes
>
> + ASPIRIN > 160 mg orally every day (chewable is preferred for first dose)
>
> + HEPARIN (5000 U bolus followed by 1000 U/hour; aPTT = 60 to 85 seconds

The recommendations for acute MI with thrombolysis are based primarily on the results of the Global Utilization of Streptokinase and Tissue Plasminogen Activator for Occluded Coronary Arteries (GUSTO I) trial (14). In this study of 41,021 patients, the use of recombinant tPA was associated with fewer deaths in comparison to SK: the 30-day mortality was 6.3% with tPA versus 7.4% with SK. tPA, however, was associated with a small increased rate of hemorrhagic strokes (the most serious bleeding complication of thrombolytic therapy): 0.72% with tPA versus 0.54% with SK. A combined end point of death or disabling stroke was observed in 6.9% of the tPA group and 7.8% of the SK group ($P = .006$).

Other thrombolytics currently available for intravenous administration for patients with MI are SK (1,500,000 units given over a 1-hour infusion), APSAC (anisoylated plasminogen-streptokinase activator complex; anistreplase; 30 units in a single intravenous injection over 5 minutes), and reteplase (Retavase; 10 U bolus, repeated 30 minutes later) (see Chapter 8). APSAC is a chemically modified SK in which the active site of plasminogen is acylated and then complexed to SK. APSAC undergoes slow spontaneous deacylation in vivo, resulting in plasmin-generating activity that is relatively resistant to endogenous plasmin inhibitors. Reteplase is a mutant tPA molecule in which a large region of the protein is deleted. This results in a longer serum half-life, and effective thrombolysis can be achieved with two bolus injections 30 minutes apart; this suggests that reteplase may be useful in treating acute MI in patients before they reach the hospital.

Each of these agents catalyzes the conversion of plasminogen to plasmin. They have different half-lives: SK about 23 minutes; APSAC about 90 minutes; reteplase about 15 minutes; and tPA initially about 4 minutes. tPA is relatively specific for deposited fibrin, leading to a two-phase pharmacokinetic profile with a terminal half-life of about 45 minutes as bound tPA is metabolized. Neutralizing antibodies develop in patients who are given SK, so patients requiring repeat thrombolysis for MI within a year following SK should receive tPA. tPA, APSAC, and reteplase are about five times more expensive than SK (which is approximately $400 per dose).

About 50% of all patients with MI receive intravenous thrombolytic therapy, but most investigators and practitioners believe that at least three-quarters of all patients with MI should receive thrombolytics. The indications for initiating thrombolytic therapy in acute MI are ST-segment elevation (>1 mm) and a time-interval from the initiation of symptoms of less than 12 hours. Over one-half of all patients with MI do not have ST-segment elevation. Among these patients, thrombolytic therapy is recommended for patients with a new left bundle branch block, but *not* for patients with a normal ECG or ST-segment depression (15). There may also be patients who appear clinically to have a staccato pattern of coronary thrombosis; these patients may benefit from thrombolytic therapy initiated later than 12 hours following the development of symptoms. Please note that age is not a contraindication to using thrombolytics.

Bleeding occurs in about 20% of patients receiving thrombolytic therapy (with heparin and aspirin). Major bleeding (defined here as requiring a red cell transfusion) occurs in up to 10% of all patients receiving a thrombolytic agent. Hemorrhagic stroke occurs in less than 1%. The risk of bleeding has been remarkably consistent among the major studies, including GUSTO (see above), TIMI (Thrombolysis in Myocardial Infarction), and GISSI (Gruppo Italiano per lo Studio della Sopravvivenza Nell'Infarcto Miocardico) (16,17). To minimize the risk of bleeding, see the contraindications in Table 6.3.

Treatment for major bleeding associated with thrombolytic therapy is straightforward. First, stop the thrombolytic agent and heparin. If possible, apply pressure to the bleeding site. Additional measures include ε-aminocaproic

Table 6.3 Contraindications for thrombolytic therapy

Absolute Contraindications

Active internal bleeding

Intracranial neoplasm or head injury within 1 month

History of hemorrhagic stroke or recent nonhemorrhagic stroke

Suspected aortic dissection

Pregnancy

Prolonged traumatic CPR

Blood pressure reading >200/120

Trauma or surgery that is a potential bleeding source within 2 weeks

History of allergic reaction to SK or APSAC in past (for those receiving SK
  or APSAC)

Relative Contraindications

Remote stroke or TIA with complete resolution

Recent trauma or surgery >2 weeks previously

History of severe hypertension with diastolic blood pressure >120

Hemorrhagic retinopathy

Warfarin anticoagulation or bleeding diathesis

Active peptic ulcer disease

Previous treatment with SK or APSAC (does not apply to tPA)

acid (Amicar, which directly inhibits plasmin-mediated fibrinolysis), protamine (to reverse rapidly the effects of heparin), fibrinogen replacement with cryo-precipitate, and platelet transfusions (to overcome the effect of ASA). Obviously, these maneuvers are never knee-jerk, and the risk of bleeding must be measured against the risk of MI. When one decides to maintain thrombolytics plus ASA and heparin in the bleeding patient, red cell transfusions should be given to maintain the hematocrit greater than 33%.

The concomitant use of ASA and heparin with tPA is firmly established (18). How long should they be used? ASA should probably be used as long as possible—that is, as long as the patient lives. Heparin should be used for 48 to 72 hours in stable patients. In patients with evidence of ongoing or progressive ischemia, heparin should probably be continued until some additional revascularization procedure is performed. Long-term anticoagulation with warfarin is not routinely done (see below). It must be pointed out that a recent review from the United Kingdom supports the use of ASA plus SK (1,500,000 units over 1 hour), without heparin, in those patients who have not previously received SK (18).

Several new antithrombotics have been evaluated as an adjunct to thrombolytic therapy for acute MI. Results of studies employing antagonists of platelet GpIIb-IIIa (e.g., abciximab and eptifibatide) after thrombolytics are encouraging. A recently completed study (TIMI 9B) showed that the thrombin inhibitor hirudin was no more effective than unfractionated heparin when it was used in combination with thrombolytic therapy (19).

Angioplasty (with and without Stents)

Before Cardiac Catheterization
ASA 325 mg orally (chewable is preferred)

+ HEPARIN (varying doses depending on length and type of procedure)

Before Angioplasty
HEPARIN 3000 U bolus every 15 minutes (keep total dose < 20,000 U; aim for ACT of 250–300)

Abciximab (chimeric 7E3 Fab, Abciximab) 0.25 mg/kg bolus followed by 0.125 µg/kg/min (max 10 µg/min)

After Angioplasty
ASA 325 mg orally every day ad infinitum

HEPARIN (to maintain aPTT about 2 × control for hours to days)

The indications for angioplasty are difficult to simplify and the field is evolving rapidly. There are many studies demonstrating that routine angioplasty for residual stenosis after successful intravenous thrombolysis is of no benefit. On the other hand, it appears that primary angioplasty may be the optimal therapy in select patients with acute MI, including those who cannot receive thrombolytic therapy and those with cardiogenic shock or sustained hypotension (20).

Clinical investigations of antiplatelet agents that inhibit GpIIb-IIIa have mostly focused on patients receiving angioplasty (and/or stents) (21). The benefits of these therapies have been sufficiently obvious that two of them (the chimeric monoclonal antibody abciximab and the peptide eptifibatide) have been FDA-approved for use in patients at high risk. High-risk patients are those with either an acute evolving MI within 12 hours of onset; two or more episodes within 24 hours of resting chest pain with an ECG ST-segment elevation, despite optimal medical therapy for unstable angina or MI; or clinical or angiographic evidence of high-risk stenosis. Among these patients, the anti-GPIIb-IIIa agent reduced the incidence of acute ischemic events by 35% at 30 days and 26% at 6 months (22). Because some practitioners consider that only high-risk patients should receive angioplasty, the routine use of abciximab is suggested above. Please note that the dose of heparin should be decreased when abciximab is used.

Be aware that bleeding requiring treatment with red cell transfusions occurred in about 15% of patients treated with abciximab; most bleeding develops at the site of the femoral puncture and was not a life-threatening complication. There were also an unusual number of retroperitoneal hemorrhages in the treated group (12 out of 708, versus 3 of 696 for placebo). There is a small risk of treatment-related thrombocytopenia (about 2%). It is likely that bleeding complications will decrease as the optimal dose of co-administered heparin is lowered (22).

Intracoronary Stents

TICLOPIDINE 250 mg orally twice a day for 1 month

+ASA < 325 mg orally every day life-long

These recommendations are based on a study of 517 patients randomized to ticlopidine + ASA or anticoagulant therapy + ASA (23). All patients also received heparin during the angioplasty/stenting procedure. Occlusion of the stented vessel occurred in 0.8% of patients receiving dual antiplatelet therapy and 5.4% of patients receiving anticoagulant therapy with ASA. After 30 days, the antiplatelet agent arm demonstrated a substantially decreased risk of MI or need for repeat intervention (decreased by 82% and 78%, respectively). There was bleeding only in the warfarin arm of the study. Although clopidogrel is frequently substituted for ticlopidine, fewer data are available supporting its use after stenting (see Chapter 7).

Bypass Surgery

ASPIRIN 81–325 mg orally every day, to begin 6 hours after surgery

Several studies demonstrate that ASA is effective at decreasing the rate of early and late saphenous vein graft occlusion (24). When ASA is started preoperatively, there is an increased risk of bleeding, including bleeding requiring reoperation. When ASA is started more than 48 hours after surgery, the short-term occlusion rate is increased (about 15% at 10 days versus 8% in groups given ASA early after surgery). ASA is also recommended for patients who receive internal mammary artery grafts, although there are fewer studies examining antiplatelet therapies in this setting. Arterial grafts are generally preferable because they are associated with better short-term and long-term outcomes.

Ticlopidine or clopidogrel started on the second day after surgery is as effective as ASA, but its cost and side effects (including reversible neutropenia) force it into a back-up role for use in patients who fail or cannot tolerate ASA. Warfarin anticoagulation is relatively ineffective and is associated with bleeding; it is therefore not recommended.

Please be aware that cardiopulmonary bypass is associated with the development of defects in hemostasis. Most important is the onset of a markedly prolonged bleeding time related to platelet functional abnormalities caused by platelets getting activated while passing through filters and oxygenators at low temperatures. This causes a biphasic response: 1) short-term platelet hyper-reactivity contributes to graft occlusion while the patient is on the pump; and 2) there is longer term (4 to 6 days) platelet hyporeactivity due to circulating platelets that are "spent," having discharged many of their granule contents and down-regulated their adhesion receptors. Mild thrombocytopenia develops within minutes after the institution of cardiopulmonary bypass, and can last for days after the operation, contributing to the hemostatic defect. Increased fibrinolysis and mild coagulation factor deficiencies are also observed transiently (during and within about 4 hours of the completion of surgery), but their clinical significance is uncertain.

Secondary Prevention

ASPIRIN 81–325 mg orally every day

Numerous randomized placebo-controlled studies consistently demonstrate that, after MI, aspirin reduces recurrent MI and death from all vascular causes (25). The dose of ASA in most of these studies was at least 325 mg per day, and thus the lower doses recommended above are extrapolations from studies of other arterial disorders in which doses over this range are similarly effective (with lower ASA doses associated with fewer gastrointestinal toxicities). Pooled data show that for 2 years after MI, ASA eliminates 40 vascular events for 1000 at-risk persons. Age is not a contraindication for using ASA after an infarction (26).

What are the contraindications? ASA may be more harmful than beneficial in patients with bleeding (or a history of gastrointestinal bleeding), thrombocytopenia, renal insufficiency, allergy, or a history of hemorrhagic stroke. There is currently no established indication for using ASA with warfarin. Warfarin alone for about 3 months is indicated for patients with transmural anterior wall infarcts, and probably should be continued longer in patients with hypokinetic left ventricles, particularly when a mural thrombus is present. The prevention of systemic thromboembolism from a cardiac source will be discussed later in this chapter.

Cerebrovascular Thrombosis

Cerebrovascular diseases ("stroke") encompass those pathophysiologic processes resulting from brain ischemia, hypoxia, and/or hemorrhage. It is the third leading cause of death in the United States (about 150,000 per year, behind cardiovascular diseases and cancer) and the leading cause of disability (affecting about 400,000 previously functional persons annually). About 45% of all strokes, and nearly 100% of all *transient ischemic attacks* (TIAs), which is an episode of cerebrovascular ischemia lasting less than 24 hours, are due to progressive atherosclerotic narrowing in the large arteries supplying blood to the brain.

The circulation of the brain is divided in two: the anterior circulation (the internal carotid artery and its two main branches, the anterior and middle cerebral arteries) and the posterior circulation (the vertebral arteries converging to form the basilar artery). Most clinical syndromes due to atherothrombosis of the arteries supplying the brain relate to the vessel that is stenosed, and are fairly easily distinguishable at the bedside (Table 6.4). Other causes of stroke, besides atherothrombotic narrowing of the carotid or vertebrobasilar vessels, include thromboembolism from the heart (about 20%), lacunar infarcts from atherosclerotic or lipohyalinotic degeneration of small penetrating arteries (about 15%), subarachnoid hemorrhage (about 12%), and intracerebral hemorrhage

Table 6.4   Stroke syndromes

Anterior cerebral artery
- Contralateral sensorimotor deficit foot and leg > arm; face spared; + incontinence

Middle cerebral artery
- Contralateral hemiplegia and hemianesthesia (face and arm > leg), homonymous hemianopia; aphasia (dominant); impaired spatial perception (nondominant)

Posterior cerebral artery
- Isolated hemianopia or quadrantic field cut; transient global amnesia; cortical blindness (when bilateral)

Vertebrobasilar arteries
- **Wallenberg's syndrome (lateral medullary infarction):** vertigo, nausea, vomiting, nystagmus, gait and ipsilateral limb ataxia, impaired pain and temperature on ipsilateral face and contralateral body; dysphagia, hoarseness, ipsilateral palate weakness, decreased gag, Horner's syndrome and hiccups (*vertebral > posterior inferior cerebellar artery*)
- **Medial medulla:** Ipsilateral tongue weakness, contralateral weakness and decreased proprioception (*vertebral or branch of lower basilar artery*)
- **Lateral pontine:** Caudal syndrome—resembles lateral medullary syndrome (*anterior inferior cerebellar artery*); rostral syndrome—identical except cranial nerves 7 and 8 are spared (*superior cerebellar artery*)

- **Medial pontine:** contralateral hemiparesis, ipsilateral facial weakness (caudal lesions), or contralateral facial weakness (rostral lesions); ipsilateral gaze palsy; internuclear ophthalmoplegia; limb or gait ataxia; palatal myoclonus (*paramedian branches of the basilar artery*)
- **Cerebellar:** gait and limb ataxia, vomiting (*vertebral artery*)

Lacunar infarction
- Pure motor hemiplegia (*internal capsule*)
- Pure hemisensory disturbance (*thalamus*)
- Ataxic ipsilateral hemiparesis (*pons*)
- Dysarthria/clumsy hand syndrome (*caudal pons*)
- Pseudobulbar palsy: dysphagia, dysarthria, facial paralysis, impaired emotional control (*multiple frontal lobe infarcts*)

Intracerebral hemorrhage (related to hypertension)
- Putaminal (~50%): stupor or coma; hemiplegia; headache is rare
- Thalamic: hemisensory loss progressing to hemiplegia; vertical gaze palsy; unreactive pupils; headache is rare
- Pontine: rapid coma and death; total paralysis; small reactive pupils
- Cerebellar: sudden onset of nausea, vomiting, ataxia, headache
- Lobar: Localized headache; Broca's (fluent) dysphasia (*temporal lobe*); hemianopia (*occipital lobe*); contralateral hemiparesis (*frontal lobe*)

(about 5%). Lacunar infarcts and intracerebral hemorrhages are usually associated with hypertension. Their location tends to be limited to specific regions and associated with predictable clinical syndromes (see Table 6.4).

Clinical Presentation

Brain ischemia due to progressive stenosis in a cerebral artery results in a TIA or stroke. TIAs usually reflect transient arterial thromboses, and the typical TIA from atherothrombosis lasts only minutes. TIAs that last for an hour or more are often associated with embolism from a noncerebrovascular source, rather than thrombus formation upon a fixed stenosis. TIAs from retinal ischemia (that branch from the internal carotid) give a stereotypical syndrome termed *transient monocular blindness* or *amaurosis fugax*. Patients usually describe this as a shade descending over one eye. TIAs in the territory of the carotid also affect the brain supplied by the middle cerebral artery, leading to hemiparesis or hemisensory disturbances (more often of the upper extremities) and language or behavioral disturbances. Vertebrobasilar TIAs lead to a panoply of symptoms and signs, including hemiparesis, hemisensory phenomena, diplopia, vertigo, dysarthria, and ataxia.

The natural history of TIAs is sinister: 5% to 10% of untreated TIAs progress to completed stroke within 1 year. The risk is greater in patients with more frequent TIAs ("crescendo TIAs") and those with high-degree carotid stenosis; the risk is smaller in patients with amaurosis fugax. The risk continues at about 4% to 5% per year for 5 to 10 years, after which the risk approaches that of someone without a history of TIA.

A stroke results from brain infarction. The specific neurologic deficit depends on the cause of the stroke, particularly the location and magnitude of the lesion resulting in irreversible ischemia (see Table 6.4). The onset of the neurologic symptoms provides clues to the pathophysiology of a stroke syndrome. Strokes from atherothrombosis of the cerebral arteries tend to have an abrupt onset, often foreshadowed by TIAs. Cardiogenic emboli usually are of abrupt onset without preceding TIAs. Aneurysmal rupture is also abrupt in onset and rapid in progression; headache is the most common harbinger of a subarachnoid hemorrhage. In contrast, a lacunar infarct (secondary to progressive small artery narrowing from atherosclerosis and/or hypertensive vascular lipohyalinosis) tends to be associated with a staggering or step-like onset, with symptoms and signs waxing and waning ("fluctuating") over a period of up to 36 hours. Hypertensive hemorrhages also tend to be associated with a slow and smooth progression of symptoms that reach their zenith over a period generally less than 1 day.

Diagnostic Studies

Perhaps the best diagnostic study is the bedside examination, with historical details (rapidity of onset, pattern of progression, duration, and associated symptoms) and physical findings (see Table 6.4) often accurately foreshadowing the location of lesions elucidated by computed tomography (CT) or magnetic resonance imaging (MRI) scans. Diagnostic studies are also required to determine if there is intracranial blood. The presence of hemorrhage on CT scan absolutely eliminates the possibility of initiating anticoagulant or fibrinolytic therapy.

A CT scan is required to evaluate for intracerebral blood within the first 48 hours after an acute cerebrovascular event. In addition, the CT scan will image blood over the surface convexities resulting from subarachnoid hemorrhage, and identify mass lesions and pressure effects. MRI scans have greater resolution for infarction than CT scans, but this issue does not affect the immediate workup leading to therapeutic intervention in most cases. An MRI scan is very good at identifying lacunar and brain stem infarcts. MRI scans can also identify vascular lesions (i.e., aneurysms and arteriovenous malformations) larger than 4 mm.

In some situations, identifying and quantifying carotid stenosis is useful because it establishes a reliable therapeutic plan (see below). The gold standard for this is carotid angiography. Among patients with a carotid territory TIA or small stroke, those with a greater than 60–70% stenosis of the ipsilateral extracranial carotid artery benefit from carotid endarterectomy.

How does one identify these patients? Most practitioners recommend a noninvasive carotid imaging study first. Carotid duplex ultrasonography, Doppler ultrasonography, and magnetic resonance angiography are equally good at identifying carotid stenoses of 70% or greater, each demonstrating a sensitivity of about 85% and a specificity of about 98% (27). Other methods, such as the commonly used ocular impedence plethysmography, are less predictive. Patients with a positive noninvasive study who are surgical candidates should then undergo a carotid angiogram to confirm the magnitude of stenosis and optimize surgical planning.

Antithrombotic Therapies for Atherothrombotic Carotid Arterial Disease

Risk Factor Reduction

Risk factors for stroke are those listed in Table 6.1. Of particular note is smoking: quitting results in a dramatic reduction in stroke risk, such that 5 years after quitting the risk is no greater than if one had never smoked. In the past, oral contraceptive use was associated with stroke. The use of modern low-estrogen oral contraceptives is not, however, a risk factor for stroke (28).

An interesting hypothesis that has not yet been rigorously investigated is that reductions in homocysteine concentrations (with pyridoxine, folic acid, and vitamin B_{12}) could reduce the risk of stroke among the general population. This hypothesis is based on epidemiologic data that show that plasma homocysteine concentrations are directly proportional, and serum folate and pyridoxal-5'-phosphate are inversely proportional, to the prevalence of extracranial carotid artery stenosis in the elderly (29).

Primary Prevention

None

There are no interventions currently recommended for primary prevention of stroke. Regular ASA increases the risk of stroke when it is used for the primary prevention of myocardial infarction, and this remains the major caveat in recommending its use to all adults in the United States. It is important that risk factors be ranked so that primary prevention, which could some day be recommended for select patients, can be evaluated in persons who are at greatest risk (30).

Asymptomatic Stenosis

None

Although it is currently reasonable to apply the rule of thumb that only symptomatic carotid arterial diseases demand an active intervention, there is an extensive literature that describes investigations of medical and surgical therapy in asymptomatic patients with objectively demonstrated carotid stenosis (31). Why is this an important question? Obviously because it is possible that the atherosclerotic narrowing of the carotid will progress and ultimately cause a stroke. In fact, 10% of patients with asymptomatic carotid atherosclerotic vasoocclusion with stenosis between 35% and 50% who have brain CT scans demonstrate the presence of old strokes, "silent brain infarctions." In addition, the risk of stroke among persons with a 50% reduction in carotid diameter is estimated to be around 2.5% *annually.* This narrowing is identified by one of the noninvasive studies described above and measured using arteriography.

The discovery of a bruit probably warrants further analysis of the carotid anatomy with a noninvasive study, but it is, in and of itself, *a clinically meaningless physical finding.* Asymptomatic patients with carotid bruits are *not* at increased risk of stroke, even when they undergo elective surgery (32,33). Endarterectomy before a coronary artery bypass graft (CABG) for asymptomatic patients, even when there is a significant stenosis, cannot be generally recommended.

Are there better ways to manage asymptomatic individuals (with or without a bruit) who are found by a noninvasive study to have a greater than 50% stenosis? Extensive recent literature indicates that the answer is no. This does not mean, however, that better approaches will not soon emerge. The Asymptomatic Carotid Atherosclerosis Study results suggest that ASA (325 mg per day) plus risk factor reduction plus carotid endarterectomy prevents ipsilateral stroke more often than ASA plus risk reduction alone, *when the carotid stenosis is greater than 60%.*

Perhaps the most important factor affecting outcome is surgical technique and patient selection. The Veterans' Affairs Cooperative Study Group observed that carotid endarterectomy for asymptomatic stenoses greater than 50% reduced the incidence of ipsilateral stroke from 9.4% to 4.7%, but the overall outcome (stroke plus deaths) was not improved by surgery because of a larger number of cardiovascular deaths in the surgical group (34).

Although ASA alone appears not to be particularly beneficial in this group of patients (35), if a practitioner believes that something should be done, ASA is the best intervention at this time for an asymptomatic patient with a high-grade stenosis. Definitive results may yet come forth from the Asymptomatic Carotid Surgery Trial, but until then, *primum non nocere.*

TIAs and Small Strokes

ASPIRIN 81 mg orally every day

The medical management of patients who suffer from TIAs or who have had a carotid distribution stroke from which full (or near full) recovery has occurred is straightforward: aspirin (36). What is not so straightforward is the optimal dose. Aspirin dosing for patients with symptomatic carotid arterial stenosis can be as complex as one wants to make it.

There are not, however, any convincing arguments that it needs to be complex. As Patrono and Roth note, "until additional information from ongoing clinical trials is available, good clinical practice should dictate the use of the lowest dose of aspirin shown effective in the prevention of stroke and death in patients with ischemic cerebrovascular disease" (37). The minimum effective dose is 30 mg daily (38), but this preparation is harder to find than a baby aspirin (81 mg).

For those who cannot tolerate ASA or whose pattern of TIAs does not improve with ASA, 250 mg of ticlopidine orally twice a day or 75 mg of clopidogrel orally every day is the treatment of choice for preventing stroke (39). Although one study demonstrated that ticlopidine was somewhat more effective than ASA, its use is associated with far more side effects, including diarrhea (20%), rash (14%), and severe reversible neutropenia (1%). Clopidogrel has fewer side effects, but its beneficial effects have not been established as extensively as have ticlopidine's (see Chapter 7). The risk of minor bleeding with these agents is about the same as with ASA (about 10% of patients).

Symptomatic 70% Carotid Stenosis

Endarterectomy
+ ASA 81 mg per day

The benefit of surgical removal of atherosclerotic plaque in patients with TIAs or prior small (nondisabling) strokes is firmly established when the arterial narrowing involves at least 70% of the luminal diameter. The stenosis must be defined by arteriography, although a noninvasive study is usually performed first to select the patients likely to fulfill the arteriography criteria of surgical intervention. Almost all patients receive concomitant ASA, although one controlled study suggested that this does not prevent restenosis and might actually worsen outcome (40).

How good is endarterectomy for symptomatic patients with greater than 70% stenosis? Very good: among 328 patients who received this procedure the risk of ipsilateral stroke at 2 years was 9%, versus 26% in the nonsurgical group (treated with risk factor reduction plus ASA). Mortality from stroke was decreased from 13.1% to 2.5% in the surgical group (41). The benefit of endarterectomy in patients with less than 70% but greater than 50% stenosis is less (42).

How risky is endarterectomy? In one study, the short-term (perioperative) risk for death or disabling stroke, which extends for about 1 month, was 0.6% and 2.1%, respectively, in the surgical group; it was 0.3% and 0.9%, respectively, in the nonsurgical group (41). It is advisable that one scrutinize patient outcomes for institutions and individual surgeons before recommending endarterectomy (42).

Acute Atherothrombotic Stroke

CT Scan (–) for Bleeding or Swelling; within 3 Hours of Onset

Intravenous tPA to a total dose of 0.9 mg/kg (maximum 90 mg)

10% dose bolus followed by a 60-minute infusion of the remaining 90%

Exclusion criteria

1. Use of anticoagulants, PT > 15 seconds, or INR > 1.7
2. Use of heparin within 48 hours and a prolonged aPTT
3. Platelets < 100,000/µl
4. Another stroke or serious head injury within 3 months
5. Major surgery within 14 days
6. Pretreatment blood pressure, diastolic > 110 or systolic > 185 mm Hg
7. Rapidly improving neurologic signs
8. Isolated, mild neurologic deficits (e.g., ataxia, sensory loss alone, dysarthria alone, or minimal weakness)
9. Prior intracranial hemorrhage
10. Blood glucose <50 or >400 mg/dL
11. Seizure at stroke onset
12. Gastrointestinal or urinary bleeding within 21 days
13. Recent MI

Although this approach has not yet gained widespread acceptance, the therapeutic index is clearly established when the patients are properly selected. It is suggested that a multidisciplinary team approach be initiated to develop and support a system for gathering the benefits of this approach. And what are those benefits? Of 333 patients randomized to tPA or placebo, those given tPA were observed to be at least 30% more likely to have minimal or no disability at 3 months (43). Symptomatic intracranial hemorrhage within 36 hours of the onset of the stroke (despite careful selection) occurred in 6.4% of those given tPA and 0.6% of those receiving placebo. Mortality at 3 months was 17% in the tPA group and 21% in the placebo group (not a significant difference). Other thrombolytic therapies cannot be currently recommended (2). Because of the risk of hemorrhage, tPA therapy should be thoroughly discussed with patients and family members. Despite sustained benefits having been demonstrated, thrombolytic therapy for acute stroke remains a controversial intervention (44,45).

CT Scan (–) for Bleeding or Swelling; > 3 Hours after Onset

Unfractionated heparin 5000 U subcutaneous twice a day or three times a day; or

Low-molecular-weight heparin (e.g., enoxaparin, 30 mg subcutaneously twice a day)

Prophylactic doses of heparin are clearly beneficial at preventing venous thromboembolism, including mortality from pulmonary embolism, among patients with ischemic strokes who have no hemorrhage on CT. For those who have hemorrhage, mechanical devices such as graduated elastic compression stockings or intermittent pneumatic compression should be used to prevent DVT, although they are not as effective as heperin (46). A recent study suggests that therapeutic doses of low-molecular-weight heparin (LMWH) may be beneficial in this group, although confirmation in a larger number of patients will be required before this becomes the standard of care (47).

What about concern that a "bland infarct" will become hemorrhagic and cause neurologic deterioration? In fact, most studies that have looked for this have failed to find an increase above controls, observing 6% to 7% hemorrhagic transformation on CT scanning 14 days after the acute event whether or not heparin was used. Even when full-dose LMWH was used there was no statistically significant increase in hemorrhage into the ischemic brain on CT scans performed 10 days after presentation: 6.2% in the full-dose group versus 8.6% in the prophylactic dose group versus 12% in the placebo group (47).

Antithrombotic Therapies for Cardiogenic Stroke

Cardiogenic strokes arise within three clinical settings: atrial fibrillation; artificial heart valves, and left ventricular mural thrombosis.

Atrial Fibrillation

Primary Prevention: High-risk Patients

WARFARIN (INR 2.0–3.0)
>   Mitral stenosis
>   Hypertension
>   Prior stroke or TIA
>   Diabetes
>   Recent heart failure
>   Age > 65 years

Primary Prevention: Low-risk Patients

ASPIRIN 325 mg/day
None of the above ("lone atrial fibrillation")

The major concern with the direct implementation of such treatment programs is the risk of bleeding among older patients taking warfarin. This risk is real, but controllable with careful monitoring of the INR. In elderly patients who cannot tolerate warfarin (perhaps as many as one-third), ASA is an acceptable, although inferior, alternative primary prevention (48).

What are the benefits of primary prevention with warfarin at the targeted INR in patients with chronic or intermittent atrial fibrillation? There is a reduction by at least 50% in the incidence of strokes, which ranges from 5% to 7% per year in untreated persons. Aspirin is about one-half as effective as warfarin (49). What are the risks? In the study of secondary prevention with warfarin, bleeding developed in only 2 of 186 patients whose INR was maintained in the 2.0–2.9 range, and the bleeding was age independent (50).

Secondary Prevention
WARFARIN (targeted to INR of 2.0–3.0)

Start medication about 1 week after acute stroke

This treatment decreases the risk of recurrent cerebral thromboembolism (about 10% per year in untreated patients) by around two-thirds. Warfarin does not work with an INR < 2.0, and the bleeding risk increases substantially at an INR > 4.0. ASA is a less effective alternative for patients who do not tolerate warfarin. Of note is that recurrence rarely occurs within 2 weeks, so slow initiation of warfarin (without heparin) can be used in this setting (50).

One important consideration in managing patients with chronic/intermittent atrial fibrillation who have had a stroke or TIA is the possibility that the cerebral ischemic event is secondary to carotid stenosis rather than embolism from an atrial thrombus. About 15% of patients with stroke and associated atrial fibrillation have ipsilateral carotid stenosis. In patients with ipsilateral stenosis greater than 70%, a transesophageal echocardiogram is recommended to exclude atrial thrombosis before endarterectomy is performed. In the patient with both atrial thrombus and carotid stenosis, warfarin remains the treatment of choice.

Cardioversion of Atrial Fibrillation
WARFARIN (for 3 weeks before and 4 weeks after cardioversion; target INR 2.0–3.0)

These are the recommendations of the American Heart Association (48). Two modifications may be useful. When patients have atrial fibrillation of less than 48 hours' duration or are clinically unstable, it may be reasonable to administer full-dose heparin, cardiovert when the aPTT is about 2 × control, and continue warfarin anticoagulation for 4 weeks. Similarly, in patients with longer or unknown duration atrial fibrillation who are clinically stable, recent evidence suggests that the duration of anticoagulant therapy can be shortened with the use of a transesophageal echocardiogram (TEE) (51). A TEE that shows no atrial thrombus directs a patient to full heparinization followed by immediate cardioversion. When this is successful, warfarin is continued for 4 additional weeks.

What is the usual outcome using the standard approach? The prevalence of cardioversion-related cerebral thromboembolism is decreased from 5% to 1%, and between 70% to 80% of patients will be in sinus rhythm at the 4-week time point, allowing for the discontinuation of warfarin (52).

Prosthetic Heart Valves

Warfarin anticoagulation is used chronically in patients with mechanical valves and for 3 months after placement of a bioprosthetic heterograft (53). In general, mechanical valves require relatively intensive anticoagulation, although the intensity is adjusted depending on the type of mechanical valve.

Caged Ball or Multiple Mechanical Valves
WARFARIN (targeted to INR 4.0–4.9)

Single Tilting Disc Valves
WARFARIN (targeted to INR 3.0–3.9)

Bileaflet Disc Valves
WARFARIN (targeted to INR 2.0–2.9)

Bioprosthetic Valves
WARFARIN (targeted to INR 2.0–3.0) for 3 months

The warfarin should be started within 12 hours of the surgery. Using these programs, the incidence of adverse events (thromboembolic stroke or bleeding) is kept below 3 per 100 patient years. In patients with atrial fibrillation or recurrent thromboembolism, daily aspirin (100 mg) plus warfarin (INR 3.0–4.5) should be used (54). Patients who need surgery should have the warfarin stopped about 5 days before the operation; should be placed on heparin until the time of surgery; and then should have heparin followed by warfarin, resumed as soon as possible after the surgery (see Chapter 19).

Patients with prosthetic valve endocarditis can be maintained on routine anticoagulation. If they suffer a cerebral embolic event, management depends upon the results of the brain CT scan: if no hemorrhage is present, warfarin should be continued; if hemorrhage is observed, warfarin should be stopped for 7 to 14 days and then restarted at full dose (55).

Left Ventricular Mural Thrombus

WARFARIN (INR 2.0–3.0) for 3 to 4 months

As discussed earlier, 3 months of warfarin anticoagulation may decrease systemic thromboembolism among patients with transmural anterior wall MI. This is probably due to the frequent association of a left ventricular mural thrombus with anterior wall MI (about one-third of patients) (56).

Management of Other Stroke Syndromes

There are no specific interventions for lacunar infarcts. Hypertensive hemorrhages should be managed with antihypertensive therapy and, sometimes, neurosurgical evacuation. Intracranial aneurysms are a significant public health problem, with rupture occurring in about 1 out of 10,000 persons in the United States (fatal in over one-half) and asymptomatic (and undiagnosed) aneurysms affecting at least 1 million persons (57).

Intracranial Bleeding

Reverse coagulopathy
Neurosurgical consultation
Control hypertension
DVT prophylaxis with intermittent pneumatic compression

Blacks have twice the risk of subarachnoid hemorrhage than whites. Patients with polycystic kidney disease, a family history of cerebral aneurysms, or previous aneurysms should be screened with MRI angiography for the presence of asymptomatic aneurysms. These occur in up to 10% of such populations, and the risk of rupture may approach 6 per 10,000 persons per year. Surgery is the primary management for an asymptomatic or ruptured aneurysm. Patients with a ruptured aneurysm should receive the calcium antagonist nimodipine intravenously to prevent vasospasm. Antifibrinolytic therapy (e.g., ε-aminocaproic acid or tranexamic acid) is not recommended. Although it decreases aneurysmal bleeding, it enhances ischemia and worsens infarction, thus resulting in no net therapeutic benefit.

Strokes of Unknown Origin

Diagnostic considerations (younger patients without obvious cause)

1. paradoxical embolism (contrast echocardiography)
2. atheroembolism from aortic arch (transesophageal echocardiogram)
3. cocaine use (urine toxicology screen)

Paradoxical embolism through a patent foramen ovale can cause stroke (58). In at least 20% of the general population, a patent foramen ovale is observed by contrast echocardiography ("bubble study") (59). This may increase the risk of stroke, and it is reasonable to look for a patent foramen ovale in a stroke patient of any age who lacks an obvious cause for the stroke. Paradoxical embolism is treated with routine anticoagulation or an interior vena cava (IVC) filter.

Another diagnostic consideration in patients without any clear origin for cerebral ischemic infarction is an ulcerated plaque in the aortic arch. This is diagnosed by transesophageal echocardiography. One study demonstrated the presence of atherosclerotic plaques greater than 4 mm in 14.4% of stroke patients versus 2% of normal controls (60). Another group related a 30% yearly incidence of embolism when the aortic plaque includes protruding atheromata, intimal ulceration, or mobile thrombi (61). Thrombolysis and surgical removal have been used to treat associated embolism, but neither these nor any other treatments are predictably effective. Surgical thromboembolectomy ("aortic endarterectomy") is a technically feasible means of preventing recurrence in high-risk patients. Currently, there are no clear-cut indications or outcomes for this procedure, although it should be considered in patients with recurrence who are good surgical candidates. Warfarin may be beneficial in patients with pedunculated and mobile elements within the atherosclerotic plaque. There is currently no information about aspirin in this setting. Extrapolating from clinical studies of coronary and carotid stenosis, I recommend that patients in whom no other intervention is feasible or safe take one baby aspirin per day.

In an urban population, 47% of all strokes that occurred in young persons (ages 15 to 44) were related directly to cocaine use or drug abuse–associated endocarditis (62).

Peripheral Artery Thrombosis

Clinical Presentation

Claudication resulting from peripheral arterial disease (PAD) of the aorta and its downstream ilial, femoral, and popliteal branches affects over 5% of men between the ages of 55 and 64, with the yearly incidence rising with increasing age to over 7% for those over 70. The risk for women ages 64 and greater is nearly the same as the risk for men (63). The natural history of PAD is somewhat predictable: about three-fourths of patients with PAD who survive for several years after diagnosis will have stable disease, while the remaining one-quarter will have deterioration and 1% to 5% eventually will require amputation.

Beside the morbidity related to PAD, PAD is associated with severe CAD in about 60% of persons. PAD is therefore a surrogate for mortality risk related to CAD. One study determined that there was a 15-fold increase in 10-year mortality from CAD for patients with large-vessel PAD (64).

Arterial occlusion resulting in change in the clinical state of a limb can be acute (often caused by an embolism) or chronic (usually caused by progressive stenosis). In both cases, occlusion develops in an artery that is affected by atherosclerosis, and the rate of change of symptoms and signs directs one to the triggering event and its potential treatments. Chronic vasoocclusion is usually associated with claudication that, when related to aortoiliac disease, involves the buttock, thigh, or calf. There may be associated sexual dysfunction and tissue ulceration. Acute vasoocclusion results in extremity coolness, cyanosis, and pain, sometimes associated with nerve dysfunction and gangrene, and sometimes relieved by dangling the affected leg. In both cases, the pulses are decreased or absent, there is poor capillary refill, and there may be signs of chronic ischemia such as skin atrophy, hair loss, pallor, and a cold temperature. Another clinical manifestation is renal insufficiency. Atheroembolism involving the renal branches of the aorta has been reported to cause between 5% and 10% of all acute renal failure cases, so watch out for this in PAD patients who develop deteriorating renal function (65).

Diagnostic Studies

The presence and magnitude of PAD can be measured by a variety of noninvasive studies. These generally remain "second-string" studies in comparison to arteriography, but are useful for diagnosis in patients for whom surgical intervention is not an immediate concern.

Most patients with acute arterial occlusion probably require arteriography to establish the site and source of the stenosis and to plan an effective early therapeutic intervention. One possible exception to this is the use of MRI angiography. In one investigation it proved comparable to dye arteriography in identifying the lesion and actually superior to a dye study in identifying distal runoff vessels likely to accommodate bypass grafting (i.e., it directed a limb-sparing procedure) (66).

Duplex ultrasonography is excellent at measuring flow in the aortoiliac and femoropopliteal systems, and can also quantify the thickness of atherosclerotic plaque in the common femoral artery. Doppler segmental pressure measurements that reveal a greater than 30 mm Hg pressure differential between upstream and downstream segments are diagnostic of a significant occlusion. Less accurate pressure differential measurements are obtained by measuring thigh and calf blood pressure using sphygmomanometry.

Antithrombotic Therapies for Atherothrombotic Peripheral Vascular Diseases

Currently, PAD is mainly a surgical disease. In most cases, its treatment involves surgical bypass with synthetic graft materials, although a harvested saphenous vein is sometimes used for femoropopliteal bypass grafting. Balloon angioplasty is increasingly used for patients with specific types of anatomic defects (discrete stenoses), and a variety of endarterectomy procedures are becoming available.

In considering medical interventions for patients with PAD two principles prevail: 1) there are far fewer data to support concrete recommendations for treatment of patients with PAD than are available for planning treatments for patients with CAD and carotid arterial diseases, and 2) in the absence of good clinical data, treatment decisions are often based on the assumption that what works for CAD or stroke probably will work for PAD. Future work in this field should correct the former and measure the validity of the latter of these principles.

Primary Prevention

> None

Like stroke, there are no specific interventions to prevent the development of PAD. Although presently unproven, it is possible that there may be a preventive effect of ASA. In the Physicians' Health Study, there were substantially fewer operations for PAD in the ASA-treated group (325 mg every other day), but no decrease in the development of intermittent claudication (67).

Intermittent Claudication

> Exercise therapy
> Quit smoking
> ASA 81 mg orally every day

There are no clearly superior medical treatments for intermittent claudication. Exercise is the most important intervention. It is also important to maintain hygiene of the feet, just like in diabetic patients. If symptoms persist after 2 to 3 months, it is reasonable to try ticlopidine or clopidogrel (68) (Chapter 7). Failing this, next try 100 mg of cilostazol orally twice a day or 400 mg of pentoxifylline orally three times a day. Cilostazol and pentoxifylline appear to work by inhibiting smooth muscle cell phosphodiesterase, resulting in elevated cyclic nucleotides (cAMP and cGMP) and vasorelaxation (69). If symptoms and functional status worsen, the patients should be referred for angiography.

Aortofemoral Bypass Grafting, Stenting, Endarterectomy, or Angioplasty

HEPARIN full-dose, peri-procedure

Followed by ASA 81 mg orally every day thereafter

There are no studies that unequivocally establish the usefulness of anticoagulant or antiplatelet therapy in this situation. Almost all vascular surgeons advocate using heparin to prevent early occlusion of a stented or grafted aorta, but the optimal duration of heparin therapy is not known. In the absence of any medical therapy, the occlusion rate is about 20% to 30% at 5 years for each procedure. ASA is used to increase the patency rate, but this is speculative and based on data from coronary and carotid arteries.

Femoropopliteal Bypass Grafting, Stenting, or Angioplasty

ENOXAPARIN 60 mg subcutaneous twice a day beginning 2 hours preoperatively, and continuing for 7 days postoperatively

ENOXAPARIN 30 mg subcutaneous twice a day for 3 months

ASA 81 mg orally every day thereafter

These recommendations are an opinion, based on a randomized study of around 200 patients in which graft patency at 6 and 12 months was significantly improved by the low-molecular-weight heparin (70). This was observed in synthetic and saphenous vein graft recipients, and may reflect the inhibitory action of heparin on vascular smooth muscle cell proliferation that causes the occlusive intimal hyperplasia responsible for most graft reocclusions. Based on these data, such recommendations are extended to stented or dilated femoropopliteal arteries, but their validity in instrumented arteries remains to be established. Routine follow-up evaluations for patients who receive one of these procedures usually reveals a 70% to 90% patency rate at 5 years.

Acute Peripheral Arterial Stenosis

Full-dose heparinization

Arteriography or MRI angiography

Vascular surgery consultation

Consider catheter-directed intra-arterial urokinase

The goal of treatment for acute ischemia, usually due to embolism or atheroembolism, is limb preservation. This is a medical/surgical emergency that often taxes the resources of a system, and the skills and artistry of practitioners. The options for treatments include bypass grafting, surgical or balloon embolectomy, and the use of thrombolytics (71,72). Thrombolytics are indicated only for those patients whose limb can be maintained as viable for at least 24 hours, or for those critically ill patients for whom surgery is considered too dangerous. If neuromuscular function (of the foot, for example) is absent and there is no distal flow, thrombolytics should not be used. Thrombolytics are given by local catheter injection; systemic administration does not work. The contraindications listed above for acute MI are applied to these patients as well. Thrombolytics work best in a native vessel > synthetic graft > autologous vein graft, and in embolic rather than thrombotic occlusions. If thrombolytics have not restored adequate flow after 24 hours, an invasive or amputation procedure must be performed.

Annotated Bibliography

1. Willard JE, Lange RA, Hillis LD. The use of aspirin in ischemic heart disease. New Engl J Med 1992;327:175–181.

   A thorough review of how aspirin is used in coronary artery disease.

2. Multicentre Acute Stroke Trial-Italy (MAST-1) Group. Randomised controlled trial of streptokinase, aspirin and combination of both in treatment of acute ischaemic stroke. Lancet 1995;346:1509–1514.

   In patients with stroke, SK with or without ASA led to higher 10-day and 6-month case fatality rates than did neither drug or ASA alone. The dose of SK was 1,500,000 units infused over 1 hour administered within 6 hours of symptom onset. All patients had a brain CT scan to exclude intracerebral hemorrhage. The design of this study involved 70 centers in Europe enrolling 622 patients.

3. Coller BS. Platelets and thrombolytic therapy. New Engl J Med 1990;322:33–42.

   A classic review that bridges pathophysiology with therapeutics, by an individual who is an accomplished expert in translational basic research.

4. Steering Committee of the Physicians' Health Study Research Group. Final report on the aspirin component of the ongoing physicians' health study. New Engl J Med 1989;321:129–135.

   22,701 healthy male physicians were evaluated over an average of 5 years. They took either placebo or 325 mg of ASA every other day. The risk of MI was reduced by 44% in the ASA group, apparent only among those who were 50 years of age and older. There was a small statistically insignificant increase in the risk of hemorrhagic stroke and ulcer among the ASA users. There was no effect on overall mortality.

5. Ridker PM, Manson JE, Gaziano JM, et al. Low-dose aspirin therapy for chronic stable angina. A randomized, placebo-controlled clinical trial. Ann Intern Med 1991;114:835–839.

   The Physicians' Health Study demonstrated that ASA, 325 mg every other day, reduced the risk of first MI by 87% among male physicians with chronic stable angina.

6. Cheseboro JH, Fuster V. Thrombosis in unstable angina. New Engl J Med 1992;327:192–194.

An editorial that describes how to stratify patients with unstable angina, and some suggestions about treatments for each stratum.

7. Theroux P, Waters D, Lam J, et al. Reactivation of unstable angina after discontinuation of heparin. New Engl J Med 1992;327:141–145.

In this study, 14 of 107 patients with unstable angina whose heparin was discontinued after 6 days suffered from reactivation of unstable angina leading to MI or the need for urgent intervention. This reactivation developed within a short time following heparin being stopped (9.5 +/– 5 hours). ASA prevented reactivation following heparin discontinuation.

8. Theroux P, Kouz S, Roy L, et al. Platelet membrane receptor glycoprotein IIb/IIIa antagonism in unstable angina. The Canadian Lamifiban Study. Circulation 1996;94:899–905.

In this prospective dose-ranging double-blind study, 365 patients with unstable angina were given an infusion of lamifiban, a synthetic non-peptide GpIIb-IIIa inhibitor, for 3 to 5 days. Lamifiban protected patients from MI and death during the duration of the infusion and at 1 month. This protective effect was associated with the inhibition of ex vivo platelet aggregation and the prolongation of the bleeding times. Clinically significant bleeding was dose-related and developed only during the treatment phase (14% versus 2.2% of placebo group). The interpretation of these results is confused by the co-administration of ASA (to everyone) and heparin (to 28%). Three more recent studies of two FDA-approved agents (tirofiban and eptifibatide) strongly corroborate the conclusion that non-aspirin antiplatelet agents could become routine interventions in patients with unstable angina. (See New Engl J Med 1998;338:1488–1497. New Engl J Med 1998;338:1498–1505. New Engl J Med 1998;339:436–443.)

9. Fragmin during Instability in Coronary Artery Disease Study Group. Low molecular weight heparin during instability in coronary artery disease. Lancet 1996;347:561–568.

In this study 1506 patients were randomized to placebo or dalteparin at 120 IU/kg subcutaneously or placebo every 12 hours for 6 days, followed by daily outpatient dalteparin 7500 fIU or placebo for 35 to 40 days. The LMWH was effective in preventing MI and death (1.8% versus 4.8%) at 6 days. There was no difference at 40 or 150 days.

10. Cohen M, Demers C, Garfinkel EP, et al. A comparison of low-molecular weight heparin with unfractionated heparin for unstable coronary artery disease. New Engl J Med 1997;334:447–452.

In this randomized double-blind placebo-controlled trial of 3171 patients with rest angina, patients received either standard dose unfractionated heparin or enoxaparin at 1 mg/kg subcutaneously every 12 hours. All patients received aspirin and treatments were continued for 2 to 8 days. The composite rate of death from MI for the enoxaparin groups was 16.6% and

19.8% at 14 and 30 days, respectively; for the unfractionated heparin group the rate was 19.7% and 23.3% at 14 and 30 days, respectively. Minor bleeding occurred in 11.9% of those receiving enoxaparin and 7.2% of those receiving unfractionated heparin.

11. Hirsh J, Weitz JI. New antithrombotic agents. Lancet 1999;353:1431–1436.

    A concise review of new antiplatelet agents, LMWHs, and non-heparin thrombin inhibitors.

12. The Global Use of Strategies to Open Occluded Coronary Arteries (GUSTO) IIb Investigators. A comparison of recombinant hirudin with heparin for the treatment of acute coronary syndromes. New Engl J Med 1996;335:775–782.

    In this international study, 373 hospitals in 13 countries enrolled 12,142 patients with chest pain associated with ECG changes. Patients were randomly assigned to 72 hours of hirudin or heparin; all received ASA. Hirudin offered a small advantage (death from MI was 1.3% versus 2.1% at 24 hours, and 8.9% versus 9.8% at 30 days). There was no increased risk of bleeding complications (10% versus 8.8%).

13. ISIS-2 Collaborative Group. Randomised trial of intravenous streptokinase, oral aspirin, both, or neither among 17,187 cases of suspected acute myocardial infarction. Lancet 1988;2:349–360.

    This large study demonstrates that 160 mg per day of enteric-coated ASA reduced MI-related mortality from 11.8% to 9.4% and it is therefore the foundation for the routine practice of administering ASA in this setting.

14. The Global Use of Strategies to Open Occluded Coronary Arteries (GUSTO) Investigators. An international randomized trial comparing four thrombolytic strategies for acute myocardial infarction. New Engl J Med 1993;329:673–682.

    This study of 41,021 patients concluded that the use of recombinant tPA plus intravenous heparin was associated with fewer deaths in comparison to SK: the 30-day mortality was 6.3% with tPA plus heparin versus 7.4% with SK plus heparin. tPA, however, was associated with a small increased rate of hemorrhagic strokes (the most serious bleeding complication of thrombolytic therapy): 0.72% with tPA versus 0.54% with SK. A combined end point of death or disabling stroke was observed in 6.9% of the tPA group and 7.8% of the SK group ($P = .006$).

15. Habib GB. Current status of thrombolysis in acute myocardial infarction. Part II. Optimal utilization of thrombolysis in clinical subsets. Chest 1995;107:528–534.

    A practical summary listing specific recommendations for using thrombolytic therapy in patients who may have been previously excluded from being offered this option. *Do* offer it to elderly patients and patients with inferior wall MI or left bundle branch block. *Do not* offer it to patients with contraindications or those with a normal ECG or ST segment depression only.

16. Bovill E, Terrin ML, Stump DC, et al. Hemorrhagic events during therapy with recombinant tissue-type plasminogen activator, heparin, and aspirin for acute myocardial infarction. Results of the Thrombolysis in Myocardial Infarction (TIMI), phase II trial. Ann Intern Med 1991;115:256–265.

17. Maggioni AP, Franzosi MG, Santoro E, et al. The risk of stroke in patients with acute myocardial infarction after thrombolytic and antithrombotic treatment. Gruppo Italiano per lo Studio della Sopravvivenza nell'Infarto Miocardico II (GISSI-2), and The International Study Group. New Engl J Med 1992;327:1–6.

Bovill et al. (16) and Maggioni et al. (17), different studies conducted on different continents, show that hemorrhagic strokes occur in approximately 0.36% of patients given tPA + ASA and 0.6% of patients receiving tPA + ASA + heparin. The overall risk of bleeding was about 20% in the TIMI study, and pursuing an "invasive management strategy" with coronary angiography increases the risk of bleeding without necessarily offering any benefits.

18. Collins R, Peto R, Baiget C, Sleight P. Aspirin, heparin, and fibrinolytic therapy in suspected myocardial infarction. New Engl J Med 1997;336:847–860.

This is a review of randomized clinical trials of aspirin, of heparin, and of fibrinolytic therapy in patients with suspected acute myocardial infarction. The authors emphasize which treatments favorably affect survival and other major clinical outcomes.

19. Antman EM. Hirudin in acute myocardial infarction. Thrombolysis and Thrombin Inhibition in Myocardial Infarction (TIMI) 9B trial. Circulation 1996;94:911–921.

For this study, 2003 patients with acute MI were treated with ASA and thrombolytics (tPA or SK) and were randomized to either standard heparin or hirudin (0.1 mg/kg bolus followed by 0.1 mg/kg/hour infusion) for 96 hours to maintain an aPTT of 55 to 85 seconds. The primary end point at 30 days (death, recurrent MI, severe CHF, or cardiogenic shock) occurred in 11.9% of heparin group and 12.9% of hirudin group. There was no significant difference in bleeding complications.

20. Lange RA, Hillis LD. Immediate angioplasty for acute myocardial infarction. New Engl J Med 1993;328:726–728.

Primary angioplasty may be the optimal therapy in select patients with acute MI, including those who cannot receive thrombolytic therapy and those with cardiogenic shock or sustained hypotension.

21. Lefkovits JL, Plow EF, Topol EJ. Platelet glycoprotein IIb/IIIa receptors in cardiovascular medicine. New Engl J Med 1995;332:1553–1559.

A thorough review of the rationale and clinical experiences using agents that block the platelet receptor for fibrinogen, von Willebrand factor, vitronectin, and fibronectin. In addition to teaching about drugs that will inevitably be routinely used, evidence is presented in support of the hypothesis that these agents will break the pathogenetic cycle leading to progressive atherothrombotic vasoocclusion. Brief periods of platelet exposure to GPIIb-IIIa blockade might have long-term positive effects.

22. The EPIC [Evaluation of 7E3 for the Prevention of Ischemic Complications] Investigators. Use of monoclonal antibody directed against the platelet glycoprotein IIb/IIIa receptor in high-risk coronary angioplasty. New Engl J Med 1994;330:956–961.

    High-risk patients (those with either an acute evolving MI within 12 hours of onset; two or more episodes within 24 hours of resting chest pain with an ECG ST-segment elevation, despite optimal medical therapy for unstable angina or MI; or clinical or angiographic evidence of high-risk stenosis) were treated with the anti-GPIIb-IIIa agent abciximab. Abciximab reduced the incidence of acute ischemic events by 35% at 30 days and 26% at 6 months. Bleeding requiring treatment with red cell transfusions occurred in about 15% of patients; with most bleeding at the site of the femoral puncture. There were also an unusual number of retroperitoneal hemorrhages in the treated group (12 out of 708, versus 3 of 696 for placebo). There was also a small risk of treatment-related thrombocytopenia (about 2%).

23. Schömig A, Neumann FJ, Kastrati A, et al. A randomized comparison of antiplatelet and anticoagulant therapy after the placement of coronary-artery stents. New Engl J Med 1996;334:1084–1089.

    517 patients were randomized to ticlopidine + ASA or anticoagulant therapy + ASA after the angioplasty/stenting procedure. After 30 days, occlusion of the stented vessel occurred in 0.8% of patients receiving dual antiplatelet therapy and 5.4% of patients receiving anticoagulant therapy with ASA. After 30 days, the antiplatelet agent arm demonstrated a substantially decreased risk of MI or need for repeat intervention (decreased by 82% and 78%, respectively). There was bleeding only in the warfarin arm.

24. Nwasokwa ON. Coronary artery bypass graft disease. Ann Intern Med 1995;123:528–545.

    A detailed review of what one can expect from bypass grafts over the long-term, including a summary of interventions to optimize graft patency.

25. Antiplatelet Trialists' Collaboration. Collaborative review of randomised trials of antiplatelet therapy. I. Prevention of death, myocardial infarction, and stroke by prolonged antiplatelet therapy in various categories of patients. BMJ 1994;308:81–106.

    A must read for those who want to learn more about the "why" and "when" of aspirin's use as an antithrombotic agent.

26. Krumholz HM, Radford MJ, Ellerbeck EF, et al. Aspirin for secondary prevention after acute myocardial infarction in the elderly. Ann Intern Med 1996;124:292–298.

    An observational study demonstrating that 24% of patients over 65 years old who could receive ASA after MI, *did not* receive ASA. Increasing ASA prescriptions for these patients provides a simple means to improve their care.

27. Blakeley DD, Oddone EZ, Hasselblad V, et al. Non-invasive carotid artery testing. Ann Intern Med 1995;122:360–367.

A classic meta-analysis of the subject showing that three noninvasive procedures demonstrate great success at predicting surgically reparable carotid stenosis: duplex ultrasonography, Doppler ultrasonography, or magnetic resonance angiography. Results of B-mode ultrasonography, supraorbital ultrasonography, and oculoplethysmography correlated less well with angiographic findings.

28. Petitti DB, Sidney S, Bernstein A, et al. Stroke in users of low-dose oral contraceptives. New Engl J Med 1996;335:8–15.

Stroke is rare among women of childbearing age. Low-estrogen oral-contraceptive preparations do not appear to increase the risk of stroke.

29. Selhub J, Jacques PF, Bostom AG, et al. Association between plasma homocysteine concentrations and extracranial carotid-artery stenosis. New Engl J Med 1995;332:286–291.

The relation between the maximal degree of stenosis of the extracranial carotid arteries (as assessed by ultrasonography) and plasma homocysteine concentrations, as well as plasma concentrations and intakes of vitamins involved in homocysteine metabolism, including folate, vitamin B_{12}, and vitamin B_6, was evaluated in a cross-sectional study of 1041 elderly subjects (418 men and 623 women; age range, 67 to 96 years) from the Framingham Heart Study. The subjects were classified into two categories according to the findings in the more diseased of the two carotid vessels: stenosis of 0 to 24% and stenosis of 25 to 100%. The prevalence of carotid stenosis of > or = 25% was 43% in the men and 34% in the women. The odds ratio for stenosis of > or = 25% was 2.0 (95% confidence interval, 1.4 to 2.9) for subjects with the highest plasma homocysteine concentrations (> or = 14.4 μm per liter) as compared with those with the lowest concentrations (< or = 9.1 mumol per liter), after adjustment for sex, age, plasma high-density lipoprotein cholesterol concentration, systolic blood pressure, and smoking status (P < 0.001 for trend). Plasma concentrations of folate and pyridoxal-5'-phosphate (the coenzyme form of vitamin B_6) and the level of folate intake were inversely associated with carotid-artery stenosis after adjustment for age, sex, and other risk factors.

30. Barnett HJM, Elisz; M, Meldrum HE. Drugs and surgery in the prevention of ischemic stroke. New Engl J Med 1995;332:238–248.

This review summarizes the state of knowledge for the treatment of patients with carotid artery stenosis. The authors conclude that there is no current indication for treating patients with asymptomatic stenosis, although our knowledge base regarding this is expanding and soon it may be proven that patients with stenoses greater than 50% benefit from antiplatelet therapy.

The authors also provide an important surgical perspective and advocate carotid endarterectomy in symptomatic patients with severe stenoses.

31. Brott T, Toole JF. Medical compared with surgical treatments of asymptomatic carotid artery stenosis. Ann Intern Med 1995;123:720–722.

    The Asymptomatic Carotid Atherosclerosis Study (ACAS) results suggest that carotid endarterectomy combined with aspirin and risk factor reduction is superior to aspirin and risk factor reduction alone in preventing small ipsilateral strokes in asymptomatic patients with diameter stenosis of the carotid artery of 60% or more. The absolute strokes risk reduction over 5 years conferred by surgical therapy is modest (5.9%). For prevention of stroke in women and for prevention of major stroke, the ACAS results favoring surgery did not reach statistical significance. The combined arteriographic and perioperative surgery-related mortality and stroke rates were kept low, probably because of carefully selected surgical teams.

32. Heyman A, Wilkinson WE, Heyden S, et al. Risk of stroke in asymptomatic persons with cervical arterial bruits. New Engl J Med 1980;302:838–841.

    This is an older study surveying a rural community in Georgia, which found that 4.4% of persons over the age of 45 had cervical arterial bruits. Although the presence of the bruits appeared to reflect risks of arterial occlusive disease, and in particular coronary artery disease, it did not correlate with the risk of subsequent stroke. These authors suggest that asymptomatic cervical bruits require no specific interventions.

33. Ropper AH, Wechsler LR, Wilson LS. Carotid bruit and the risk of stroke in elective surgery. New Engl J Med 1982;307:1388–1390.

    In this study, 735 unselected patients undergoing elective surgery were examined to determine the incidence of carotid bruit and postoperative stroke. They found that 104 patients (14%) had bruits, only one of whom had a stroke within 3 days of surgery. Of the remaining 631 patients without a bruit, 4 had a stroke within 3 days after the operation. Therefore, the overall incidence of a stroke was the same in the absence or presence of the asymptomatic carotid bruits, leading to the conclusion that no specific intervention needs to be made among patients who are preparing to undergo surgery and are found to have an asymptomatic carotid bruit.

34. Hobson RW, Weiss DG, Fields WS, et al. Efficacy of carotid endarterectomy for asymptomatic carotid stenosis. The Veterans Affairs Cooperative Study Group. N Engl J Med 1993;328:221–227.

    This multicenter clinical trial at 11 Veterans Affairs medical centers studied 444 men with asymptomatic carotid stenosis shown arteriographically to reduce the diameter of the arterial lumen by 50% or more. The goal of the study was to determine the effect of carotid endarterectomy on the combined incidence of transient ischemic attack, transient monocular blindness, and stroke. The patients were randomly assigned to optimal medical treatment including antiplatelet medication (aspirin) plus carotid endarterectomy (the surgical group; 211 patients) or optimal medical treatment alone (the medical group; 233 patients). The combined incidence of ipsilateral neurologic events was 8.0% in the surgical group and 20.6% in the medical group (P < 0.001), giving a relative risk (for the surgical group vs. the medical group) of 0.38 (95% confidence interval, 0.22 to 0.67). The incidence of ipsilateral stroke alone was 4.7% in the surgical group and 9.4% in the medical group. An analysis of stroke and death combined within the first 30 postoperative days showed no significant differences. Nor were there significant differences between groups in an analysis of all strokes and deaths (surgical, 41.2%; medical, 44.2%; relative risk, 0.92; 95% confidence interval, 0.69 to 1.22). Overall mortality, including postoperative deaths, was primarily due to coronary atherosclerosis.

35. Cote R, Battista RN, Abrahamowicz M, et al. Lack of effect of aspirin in asymptomatic patients with carotid bruits and substantial carotid narrowing. The Asymptomatic Cervical Bruit Study Group. Ann Intern Med 1995;123:649–655.

    372 neurologically asymptomatic patients with carotid stenosis of 50% or more in at least one artery as determined by duplex ultrasonography were randomly assigned to receive either enteric coated aspirin, 325 mg/d, or identically appearing placebo. The duration of therapy was 2.0 years for the aspirin recipients and 1.9 years for the placebo recipients. Aspirin did not have a significant long-term protective effect in asymptomatic patients with high-grade (> or = 50%) carotid stenosis.

36. Matchar DB, McCrory DC, Barnett HJ, Feussner JR. Medical treatment for stroke prevention. Ann Intern Med 1994;121:41–53.

    An analysis of 33 publications resulted in the following suggestions. Warfarin is strongly recommended for persons with nonvalvular atrial fibrillation who are older than 60 years or who have additional risk factors for stroke. Aspirin is recommended for persons at elevated risk for bleeding when receiving warfarin. For persons with TIA or minor stroke, aspirin should be used first. Patients who do not respond to or tolerate aspirin or who have had a major stroke are reasonable candidates for ticlopidine. For patients who have had myocardial infarction, aspirin is recommended for the prevention of secondary myocardial infarction but not of stroke.

37. Patrono C, Roth GJ. Aspirin in ischemic cerebrovascular disease. How strong is the case for a different dosing regimen? Stroke 1996;27:756–760.

    A nice review by non-neurologists who are platelet experts. They effectively dissect the issue of aspirin dosing and slice through the confusing variability of dosing programs (and consequent dogma, in most cases) to offer their recommendation "to use the lowest effective dose."

38. van Gijn J, Algra A, Kapepelle J, et al. A comparison of two doses of aspirin (30 mg versus 283 mg a day) in patients after a transient ischemic attack or minor ischemic stroke. New Engl J Med 1991;325:1261–1266.

This paper compared a 30-mg with a 283-mg tablet of aspirin daily in patients who had previously suffered a TIA or a minor ischemic stroke. The study enrolled 3131 patients and the mean follow-up time was 2.6 years. In the patients taking low-dose aspirin, the frequency of death from vascular causes, nonfatal stroke, or nonfatal MI was 228 of 1555 (14.7%) as compared with 240 of 1776 (15.2%) in the higher dose group. There were 40 bleeding complications in the 30-mg group versus 53 in the higher dose group. The conclusions of the study were that 30 mg of aspirin is as effective as a 283-mg tablet of aspirin in preventing vascular events among patients who have previously suffered from a TIA or a minor ischemic stroke, and that there are fewer side effects.

39. Hass WK, Easton JD, Adams HP Jr, et al. A randomized trial comparing ticlopidine hydrochloride with aspirin for the prevention of stroke in high-risk patients. Ticlopidine Aspirin Stroke Study Group. N Engl J Med 1989;321:501–507.

    Ticlopidine was somewhat more effective than aspirin in preventing strokes. The adverse effects of aspirin included diarrhea (10%), rash (5.5%), peptic ulceration (3%), gastritis (2%), and gastrointestinal bleeding (1 percent). With ticlopidine, diarrhea (20%), skin rash (14%), and severe but reversible neutropenia (less than 1%) were noted.

40. Harker LA, Bernstein EF, Dilley RB, et al. Failure of aspirin plus dipyridamole to prevent restenosis after carotid endarterectomy. Ann Intern Med 1992;116:731–736.

    This study enrolled 163 patients, half of whom were assigned to randomly receive 325 mg of aspirin plus 75 mg of dipyridamole beginning 12 hours before surgery followed by a second dose within 8 hours of the surgery; the patients then received daily aspirin plus three times per day dipyridamole for 1 year. Half the patients received placebo medications. The results indicated that greater than 50% restenosis developed in 16% of the treated group and in 14% of the placebo group. The conclusion is that aspirin plus dipyridamole probably has no effect on restenosis for patients who undergo carotid endarterectomy.

41. North American Symptomatic Carotid Endarterectomy Trial Collaborators (NASCET). Beneficial effect of carotid endarterectomy in symptomatic patients with high-grade carotid stenosis. N Engl J Med 1991;325:445–453.

    This was a large randomized trial from 50 clinical centers throughout the United States and Canada. Patients were placed in two predetermined strata based on the severity of carotid stenosis—30 to 69% and 70 to 99%. There were 659 patients in the latter stratum. All had a hemispheric or retinal transient ischemic attack or a nondisabling stroke within the 120 days before entry and a stenosis of 70 to 99% in the symptomatic carotid artery. All received optimal medical care, including antiplatelet therapy. Life-table estimates of the cumulative risk of any ipsilateral stroke at two years were 26% in the 331 medical patients and 9% in the 328 surgical patients—for an absolute risk reduction of (+/− SE) 17 +/− 3.5%. For a major or fatal ipsilateral stroke, the corresponding estimates were 13.1% and 2.5%— an absolute risk reduction of 10.6 +/− 2.6%. Carotid endarterectomy was still found to be beneficial when all strokes and deaths were included in the analysis.

42. Chassin MR. Appropriate use of carotid endarterectomy. N Engl J Med 1998;339:1471–1472.

   This is a must-read editorial based on the NASCET report in this same issue. The paper examined the benefit of carotid endarterectomy in symptomatic patients with less severe carotid stenoses and found an absolute risk reduction of 10.1% at five years for those with stenosis of 50 to 69% but no benefit for those with stenosis of less than 50%. A prominent feature of the protocol was the inclusion only of hospitals with perioperative complication rates of 6% or less. The editorialist challenges each of us to scrutinize our institution's complication rate and make sure that the risk-benefit ratio *locally* stacks up favorably to that observed in the NASCET report.

43. Brott T, Broderick J, Kothari R, et al. Tissue plasminogen activator for acute ischemic stroke. New Engl J Med 1995;333:1581–1587.

   This breakthrough paper reported on a large long-term clinical trial in the United States involving tPA. The study was divided into two parts. Each part tested a distinct hypothesis. Part I investigated the immediate benefits of tPA among about 300 patients with acute ischemic stroke; part II studied the effect of tPA 3 months after the other treatment period. The exclusion criteria are outlined in the chapter above, and the dose of tPA was 0.9 mg per kilogram of body weight (a maximum of 90 mg), 10% of which was given as an intravenous bolus followed by delivery of the remaining 90% as a constant infusion over 60 minutes. The outcome was measured using a variety of indices and scales that attempted to objectify the neurologic status. In part I there was no significant difference between the group given tPA and the placebo group in the percentage of patients with neurologic improvement at 24 hours. In part II the long-term clinical benefit of tPA was demonstrated. As compared with patients given placebo, patients treated with tPA were at least 30% more likely to have minimal or no disability at 3 months on the various assessment scales. Asymptomatic intracerebal hemorrhage within 36 hours after the onset of stroke occurred in 6.4% of patients given tPA but in only 0.6% patients given placebo. Mortality at 3 months was 17% in the tPA group and 21% in the placebo group. The investigators concluded that, despite a clearly increased incidence of asymptomatic intracerebal hemorrhage, treatment with intravenous tPA within 3 hours of the onset of ischemic stroke improved clinical outcome at 3 months.

44. Adams HP Jr, Brott TG, Furlan AJ, et al. Guidelines for thrombolytic therapy for acute stroke: a supplement to the guidelines for the management of patients with acute ischemic stroke. A statement for healthcare professionals

from a Special Writing Group of the Stroke Council, American Heart Association. Circulation 1996;94:1167–1174.

A broad dispassionate overview of the subject based on consensus.

45. Kwiatkowski TG, Libman RB, Frankel M, et al. Effects of tissue plasminogen activator for acute ischemic stroke at one year. New Engl J Med 1999;340:1781–1787.

624 patients with stroke were randomly assigned to receive either tPA or placebo. During 12 months of follow-up, the patients with acute ischemic stroke who were treated with tPA within three hours after the onset of symptoms were more likely to have minimal or no disability compared with patients given placebo. These results indicate a sustained benefit of tPA for such patients.

46. Lowe GDO. Acute stroke. In: Hull R, Pineo GF, eds. Disorders of thrombosis. Philadelphia: WB Saunders, 1996:116–125.

A nice summary of how to provide venous thromboembolism prophylaxis to patients with acute stroke.

47. Kay R, Wong KS, Yu YL, et al. Low-molecular-weight heparin for the treatment of acute ischemic stroke. New Engl J Med 1995;333:1588–1593.

Although it is clearly established that prophylactic doses of heparin improve outcome among patients with stroke, until the time of this paper there had been no studies that objectively document the benefits of full therapeutic doses of heparin with acute ischemic stroke. This study in Hong Kong screened 2750 patients with acute stroke for enrollment; 312 patients were randomized to either full-dose LMWH or prophylactic dose LMWH administered for 10 days. The medications were begun within 48 hours of the onset of symptoms. At 6 months, 306 randomized patients were analyzed: 45% of the patients in the high-dose group, 52% of the patients in the low-dose group, and 65% of the patients in the placebo group died or became disabled. There was a significant dose-dependent effect among the three study groups in favor of LMWH. The authors concluded that among patients with ischemic stroke, treatment within 48 hours of the onset of symptoms with LMWH is effective in improving outcomes at 6 months, and that full-dose LMWH may be superior to prophylactic doses.

48. Prystowsky EN, Benson DW, Fuster V, et al. Management of patients with atrial fibrillation. Circulation 1996;93:1262–1277.

This is a comprehensive review detailing the American Heart Association recommendations for managing patients with atrial fibrillation, including the prevention of thromboembolic complications.

49. Hylek EM, Skates SJ, Sheehan MA, Singer DE. An analysis of the lowest effective intensity of prophylactic anticoagulation for patients with nonrheumatic atrial fibrillation. New Engl J Med 1996;335:540–546.

Among patients with atrial fibrillation, anticoagulant prophylaxis is effective at INRs of 2.0 or greater. Because the risk of hemorrhage rises rapidly at INRs greater than 4.0 to 5.0, tight control of anticoagulant therapy to maintain the INR between 2.0 and 3.0 is advised.

50. The European Atrial Fibrillation Trial Study Group. Optimal oral anticoagulant therapy in patients with nonrheumatic atrial fibrillation. New Engl J Med 1995;333:5–10.

   In this study of secondary prevention with warfarin, bleeding developed in only 2 of 186 patients whose INR was maintained in the 2.0–2.9 range.

51. Klein AL, Grimm RA, Black IW, et al. Cardioversion guided by transesophageal echocardiography: the ACUTE Pilot Study. A randomized, controlled trial. Assessment of Cardioversion Using Transesophageal Echocardiography. Ann Intern Med 1997;126:200–209.

   For patients with atrial fibrillation of at least two days duration, TEE-guided cardioversion with short-term anticoagulation therapy was feasible and safe. All patients were started on full-dose heparin. If no thrombus was observed, patients were immediately cardioverted and then treated with 4 weeks of warfarin (INR 2–3). Cardioversion was successful in 38/45 patients and none suffered from peripheral embolization.

52. Prytowsky EN. Management of atrial fibrillation: simplicity surrounded by controversy. Ann Intern Med 1997;126:244–246.

   This a very nice, brief editorial summarizing the current unresolved issues in managing patients with atrial fibrillation who are undergoing cardioversion. This author states that the standard approach is perfectly acceptable, but acknowledges that the use of transesophageal echocardiography may provide less expensive and equally effective protection against thromboembolism among patients with atrial fibrillation who are being cardioverted. His bottom line: "until more information is available, the method of cardioversion should be selected for each patient individually."

53. Vongatanasin W, Hillis LD, Lange RA. Prosthetic heart valves. New Engl J Med 1996;335:407–416.

   A detailed review of all issues involving prosthetic heart valves, including the provision of very specific recommendations about how thromboembolic complications of prosthetic heart valves can be managed optimally.

54. Turpie AGG, Gent M, Laupacis A, et al. A comparison of aspirin with placebo in patients treated with warfarin after heart-valve replacement. New Engl J Med 1993;239:524–529.

   This is a clinical investigation into optimizing anticoagulant therapy for patients with mechanical heart valves who are at high risk for clinical embolism. It presents a randomized double-blind placebo control study of the efficacy and safety of adding aspirin 100 mg a day to warfarin (target INR 3.0–4.5) when treating 370 patients with mechanical heart valves, or prosthetic tissue valves plus atrial fibrillation, or a history of thromboembolism. Major systemic embolism or death from vascular causes occurred in 1.9% of the aspirin-treated patients per year and in 8.5% of the placebo-treated patients per year. Major systemic embolism, nonfatal intracranial hemorrhage, or death from hemorrhage or vascular causes occurred in 3.9% of the aspirin-treated patients per year versus 9.9% of the placebo-treated patients per year. Bleeding occurred in 35% of the aspirin group as compared to 22% of the placebo group, with major bleeding occurring about the same in both groups. The conclusion of this study is that the addition of ASA to warfarin therapy reduced mortality as well as major systemic embolism in patients with mechanical heart valves and in high-risk patients with prosthetic tissue valves plus atrial fibrillation or a history of thromboembolism. Although there was some increase in bleeding, the risk of the combined treatment was more than offset by the considerable benefit.

55. Cannegieter SC, Rosendaal FR, Wintzen AR, et al. Optimal anticoagulant therapy in patients with mechanical heart valves. New Engl J Med 1995;333:11–17.

A thorough review detailing exactly how to manage patients with prosthetic heart valves.

56. Weinreich DJ, Burke JF, Pauletto FJ. Left ventricular mural thrombi complicating acute myocardial infarction. Ann Intern Med 1984;100:789–794.

A left ventricular mural thrombus was identified in one-third of the patients with an anterior wall MI.

57. Schievink WI. Intracranial aneurysms. New Engl J Med 1997;336:28–40.

This review presents just about everything that an internist needs to know about subarachnoid bleeding from intracranial aneurysms.

58. Ward R, Jones D, Haponick EF. Paradoxical embolism. Chest 1995;108:549–558.

Reviews the subject of arterial embolism from a venous thrombus that crosses into the left atrium through a patent foramen ovale.

59. McNamara RL, Lima JA, Whelton PK, Powe NR. Echocardiographic identification of cardiovascular sources of emboli to guide clinical management of stroke: a cost-effectiveness guide. Ann Intern Med 1997;127:775–787.

Transesophageal echocardiography is a cost-effective test in patients with new-onset stroke.

60. Amarenco P, Cohen A, Tzourio C, et al. Atherosclerotic disease of the aortic arch and the risk of ischemic stroke. New Engl J Med 1994;331:1474–1479.

This is the seminal paper reporting that atherosclerotic disease of the aortic arch should be regarded as a risk factor for ischemic stroke and as a possible source of cerebral emboli.

61. Kronzon I, Tunick PA. Atherosclerotic disease of the thoracic aorta: pathologic and clinical implications. Ann Intern Med 1997;126:629–637.

A thorough review of the subject. The bottom line is that protruding atherosclerotic lesions in the thoracic aorta (>4mm in thickness), with or without superimposed mobile thrombi, are an important cause of embolic disease. Transesophageal echocardiography should be considered in the work-up of patients who have unexplained embolic events involving either peripheral or cerebral arteries.

62. Kaku DA, Lowenstein DH. Emergence of recreational drug abuse as a major risk factor for stroke in young adults. Ann Intern Med 1990;113:821–827.

Among patients less than 35 years of age, drug abuse was the most commonly identified potential predisposing condition (47%), and it was the only condition with a significantly elevated relative risk for stroke (11.7). A substantial rise in the proportion of drug-related strokes was observed in the last 3 years of the study (31% in 1986 to 1988, compared with 15% in 1979 to 1985). Cocaine was the drug most frequently associated with drug-related strokes.

63. Pentecost MJ, Criqui MH, Dorros G, et al. Guidelines for peripheral percutaneous transluminal angioplasty of the abdominal aorta and lower extremity vessels. A statement for health professionals from a special writing group of the Councils on Cardiovascular Radiology, Arteriosclerosis, Cardio-Thoracic and Vascular Surgery, Clinical Cardiology, and Epidemiology and Prevention, the American Heart Association. Circulation 1994;89:511–531.

This provides a nice review of the epidemiology, pathophysiology, and treatments of PAD, including a comparison of angioplasty with bypass procedures.

64. Criqui MH, Langer RD, Fronek A, et al. Mortality over a period of ten years in patients with peripheral arterial diseases. New Engl J Med 1992;326:381–386.

This study performed two noninvasive studies on 565 men and women to establish the presence and severity of PAD. It identified 67 people with PAD, including 13 patients with severe PAD (defined by the presence of both abnormal segment to arm blood pressure ratios and abnormal flow velocities). These 67 persons were followed prospectively for 10 years. All patients with large vessel PAD had a high risk of death from cardiovascular causes (sixfold increase). In patients with severe symptomatic PAD, there was a 15-fold increase in mortality from CAD over the 10 years of follow-up evaluations.

65. Mayo RR, Schwartz RD. Redefining the incidence of clinically detectable atheroembolism. Am J Med 1996;100:524–529.

The authors surveyed inpatient nephrology consultations, and found that 99 of 402 consultations involved patients who demonstrated two or more risk factors for atheroembolism. The "substantive risk factors" were atherosclerotic cardiovascular disease, anticoagulant or thrombolytic therapy, angiography or angioplasty, vascular surgery, CPR, hypertension, hypercholesterolemia, smoking, and diabetes. Of these, 85 records were reviewed; 11 supported a probable diagnosis of atheroembolism. Three out of four members of this group that were studied had pathologic confirmation of atheroembolism.

66. Owen RS, Carpenter JP, Baum RA, et al. Magnetic resonance imaging of angiographically occult runoff vessels in peripheral arterial occlusive disease. New Engl J Med 1992;326:1577–1581.

    MR angiography has a greater sensitivity for detecting distal runoff vessels and is less invasive than conventional contrast angiography. It may be better at guiding a surgeon to effective arterial reconstruction, thereby salvaging ischemic limbs.

67. Goldhaber SZ, Manson JE, Stampfer MJ, et al. Low-dose aspirin and subsequent peripheral artery surgery in the Physicians' Health Study. Lancet 1992;340:143–145.

    Among 22,071 healthy U.S. male physicians aged 40–84, there were, during an average of 60.2 months of treatment and follow-up, 56 participants who underwent peripheral arterial surgery (20 took aspirin 325 mg every other day, 36 received placebo). The relative risk of peripheral artery surgery in the aspirin group was 0.54 (P = 0.03). These data indicate that chronic administration of low-dose aspirin to apparently healthy men reduced the need for peripheral arterial surgery.

68. Blasano F, Coccheri S, Libretti A, et al. Ticlopidine in the treatment of intermittent claudication: a 12 month double-blind trial. J Lab Clin Med 1989;114:84–91.

    This reasonably well-controlled study concludes that ticlopidine 250 mg po bid improves blood flow and limb function in a small group of persons suffering from intermittent claudication.

69. Dawson DL, Cutler BS, Hiatt WR, et al. A comparison of cilostazol and pentoxifylline for treating intermittent claudication. Am J Med 2000;109:523–530.

    In this study, 698 patients with moderate to severe claudication were randomized to receive either cilostazol (100 mg orally, twice a day) or pentoxifylline (400 mg orally, twice a day). Maximal walking distance was measured at frequent intervals up to 24 weeks after beginning treatment. There was a 54% increase in walking distance in the cilostazol group (a mean of 107 meters), a 30% increase (64 meters) in the pentoxifylline group, and a 34% increase (65 meters) in the placebo group. The increase in the walking distance among the cilostazol-treated patients was statistically significant, but the protocol was accompanied by more side effects (headaches, palpitations, and diarrhea).

70. Edmondson RA, Cohen AT, Das SK, et al. Low-molecular-weight heparin versus aspirin and dipyridamole after femoropopliteal bypass grafting. Lancet 1994;344:914–918.

LMWH was better than aspirin and dipyridamole in maintaining femoropopliteal-graft patency in patients with critical limb ischemia undergoing salvage surgery.

71. Berridge DC, Gregson RH, Hopkinson BR, Makin GS. Randomized trial of intra-arterial recombinant tissue plasminogen activator, intravenous recombinant tissue plasminogen activator and intra-arterial streptokinase in peripheral arterial thrombolysis. Br J Surg 1991;78:988–995.

Sixty patients were recruited into a randomized parallel group comparison of three thrombolytic regimens for acute or subacute peripheral arterial thrombosis. There were no significant differences in age, duration of occlusion, or presence of neurosensory deficit between the groups. Initially successful lysis was significantly greater with intraarterial (IA) recombinant tissue plasminogen activator (tPA) than with either IA streptokinase (SK) or intravenous (IV) tPA. Limb salvage at 30 days was achieved in 80%, 60%, and 45%, respectively, for IA tPA, IA SK, and IV tPA. Hemorrhagic complications occurred in six patients following IA SK and in 13 following IV tPA, but only one minor hemorrhage occurred following a catheter perforation in a patient who received IA tPA.

72. Ouriel K, Veith FJ, Sasahara AA. A comparison of recombinant urokinase with vascular surgery as initial treatment for acute arterial occlusion of the legs. Thrombolysis or Peripheral Arterial Surgery (TOPAS) Investigators. New Engl J Med 1998;338:1105–1111.

This randomized, multicenter trial conducted at 113 North American and European sites compared vascular surgery (e.g., thrombectomy or bypass surgery) with thrombolysis by catheter-directed intraarterial recombinant urokinase; all patients (272 per group) had suffered acute arterial obstruction of the legs for 14 days or less. Infusions were limited to a period of 48 hours (mean of 24 hours), after which lesions were corrected by surgery or angioplasty if needed. The primary end point was the amputation-free survival rate at 6 months. Angiograms, which were available for 246 patients treated with urokinase, revealed recanalization in 196 (79%) and complete dissolution of thrombus in 167 (68%). Both treatment groups had similar significant improvements in mean ankle-brachial blood-pressure index. Amputation-free survival rates in the urokinase group were 71.8% at 6 months and 65.0% at 1 year, as compared with respective rates of 74.8% and 69.9% in the surgery group (P > 0.2). At 6 months the surgery group had undergone 551 open operative procedures (excluding amputations), as compared with 315 in the thrombolysis group. Major hemorrhage occurred in 32 patients in the urokinase group (12.5%) as compared with 14 patients in the surgery group (5.5%) (P = 0.005). There were four episodes of intracranial hemorrhage in the urokinase group (1.6%), one of which was fatal, but no episodes of intracranial hemorrhage in the surgery group.

7

Antiplatelet Agents

Platelets trigger arterial thrombosis developing in the setting of arterial injury, particularly acute injury superimposed on chronic atherosclerotic vascular disease. The trigger begins with platelet activation. Platelet activation can be initiated by many stimuli, but most initiating stimuli converge on just a few biochemical pathways that lead to important functional responses. The classic antiplatelet agent aspirin was used long before its mechanism of action was discovered. Nonetheless, it remains the only clinically useful antiplatelet agent that works by blocking an intracellular metabolic pathway leading to the synthesis of thromboxane A_2 (TXA_2), a proaggregatory and vasoconstricting product. Among the new agents in use to treat platelet-dependent thrombosis, some have been designed rationally (the GpIIb-IIIa blockers abciximab and eptifibatide), and others were discovered serendipitously (ticlopidine) and then chemically modified to improve the therapeutic index (clopidogrel) despite an incomplete understanding of the mechanism of action. The most potent of these antiplatelet agents target a cell surface response that is a final common pathway for platelet thrombus formation: the binding of fibrinogen to GpIIb-IIIa leading to platelet aggregation. The inhibition of this final common pathway has a profound effect on hemostasis, and can lead to major bleeding complications (1). The future of antiplatelet pharmacology will focus on developing drugs that inhibit thrombosis while maintaining, to whatever extent possible, platelet-dependent hemostasis.

The Molecular Basis of Antiplatelet Therapy

Figure 7.1 schematizes the three phases of platelet function: adhesion, release (or secretion), and aggregation. Each phase involves specific molecular interactions or responses, which could be targets of pharmacologic intervention.

Phase 1: Adhesion

The adhesion reaction effecting thrombosis involves platelets binding to vessel wall collagen and von Willebrand factor (vWF). The receptors that mediate

Adhesion ("Trigger")

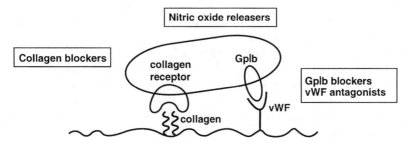

Release ("Amplification and Recruitment")

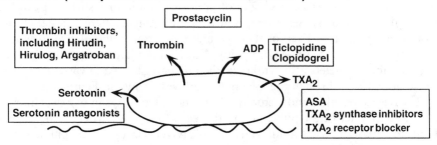

Aggregation ("Final Common Pathway")

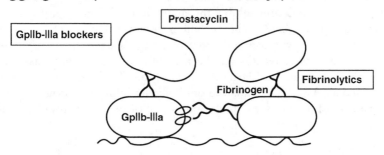

Figure 7.1. Antiplatelet agents and their mechanisms of action. (Reproduced with permission from Loscalzo J, Schafer AI, eds. Thrombosis and hemorrhage. 2nd ed. Philadelphia: Lippincott Williams & Wilkins, 1998. Copyright ©1998, Lippincott Williams & Wilkins Co.)

adhesion include several collagen-binding platelet surface molecules, the most important of which may be the integrin $\alpha_2\beta_1$, and the vWF receptor designated the GpIb/IX/V complex. The GpIb/IX/V complex binds to vWF that is in a solid phase within the subendothelium of the vessel wall, and it binds to plasma vWF that attaches to collagen exposed when the vessel wall is damaged. Under flow conditions present in narrowed arteries, platelet GpIb/IX/V binding to vWF is the *sine qua non* of platelet thrombosis, mediating the initial attachment and triggering activation resulting in release and aggregation. The direct attachment of platelets to collagen via $\alpha_2\beta_1$ plays a key supporting role in the adhesion reaction. Currently, there are no drugs available that target these molecular interactions. Although nitrates and other compounds related to nitric oxide cause elevated levels of platelet cytosolic cyclic GMP and inhibit the adhesion reaction in vitro, they are not very potent inhibitors and they have not been proven to be clinically useful for inhibiting platelet-dependent thrombosis in humans.

Phase 2: Release

Activated platelets release a variety of preformed molecules such as thrombin (from alpha granules), serotonin, and adenosine diphosphate (the latter two from dense granules). Each of these stimuli binds to specific platelet receptors and causes activation, thereby recruiting circulating platelets into the developing thrombus. Platelets also synthesize the proaggregatory and vasoconstricting prostanoid TXA_2 through the metabolic pathway shown in Figure 7.2.

The release reaction and virtually all metabolic pathways in platelets (including those that activate GpIIb-IIIa) are turned off by prostacyclin (PGI_2), which binds to a platelet receptor and activates adenylyl cyclase, resulting in increased cytosolic cyclic AMP. Unfortunately, the therapeutic index of infused PGI_2 precludes its use in humans (it causes profound hypotension) and oral PGI_2 is poorly absorbed with no significant effects on the circulating platelets among those taking it as an antacid medication.

Ticlopidine and clopidogrel inhibit the activation of platelets by released adenosine diphosphate (ADP). The thrombin receptor inhibitors, serotonin antagonists, and TXA_2 synthase and receptor blockers have all been studied in humans, but their effectiveness has been insufficient to warrant fast-track approval by the U.S. Food and Drug Administration. To date, none are commercially available. Aspirin remains the only platelet-inhibiting drug available whose mechanism of action is the inhibition of one of the pathways of platelet release.

Phase 3: Aggregation

Aggregation results in a clump of platelets that plugs the lumen of the blood vessel and causes downstream ischemia or infarction. Aggregation is caused by the cohesive interplatelet binding that bridges fibrinogen and/or vWF to adjacent platelets. Fibrinogen and vWF glue the platelets together, and each attaches to points on the platelet surface that are identified as the activated GpIIb-IIIa complex. Phase 3 therefore requires that the platelet become activated so that the GpIIb-IIIa complex is switched "on" into a conformation that permits binding to fibrinogen and vWF.

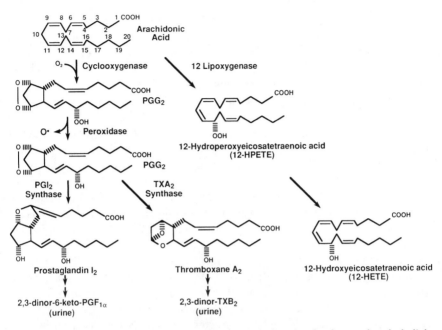

Figure 7.2. Pathways of arachidonic acid (AA) metabolism in platelets and endothelial cells. AA is liberated from membrane phospholipid and converted by prostaglandin (PG) G_2/H_2 synthase to prostaglandin endoperoxides (cyclooxygenase pathway). This pathway is inhibited by aspirin. The endoperoxides are then metabolized in different cells to products with opposite functions: platelet thromboxane A_2 (TXA$_2$) is proaggregatory and vasoconstricting, whereas endothelial cell prostacyclin (PGI$_2$) is antiaggregatory and vasodilatory. These eicosanoids are then nonenzymatically metabolized to stable 2,3-dinor end products. Platelets also contain 12-lipoxygenase that converts AA to 12-HETE, the function of which is uncertain. (Reproduced with permission from Loscalzo J, Schafer AI, eds. Thrombosis and hemorrhage. 2nd ed. Philadelphia: Lippincott Williams & Wilkins, 1998. Copyright ©1998, Lippincott Williams & Wilkins Co.)

The drugs that are used to block this final common pathway work by binding to activated GpIIb-IIIa and preventing the binding of the cohesive ligand. Fibrinolytic agents (Chapter 8) digest the fibrinogen and vWF bridges, and this effect may contribute to their efficacy in treating arterial thrombotic disorders.

FDA-Approved Antiplatelet Agents

Aspirin

Aspirin (acetylsalicylic acid) irreversibly acetylates a key enzyme in the pathway responsible for the synthesis of TXA$_2$. The enzyme functions as a cyclooxygenase (see Fig. 7.2), and is one subunit of the enzyme complex designated prostaglandin (PG) G/H$_2$ synthase or COX-1. The acetylation of this enzyme inhibits the conversion of arachidonic acid to TXA$_2$, and this block continues throughout the life span of the aspirinated platelets (about 10 days). Figure 7.1 shows that aspirin will also block the synthesis of PGI$_2$ (prostacyclin), which is synthesized by the vascular endothelium and is a potent vasodilator and anti-aggregatory prostaglandin. These latter effects are counterproductive for persons with arterial thrombosis, but the effect of aspirin on the vascular endothelium is minimized by low doses of aspirin (80 mg or less per day) (2). This is the basis for the recommendation that whenever aspirin is being used, that it be used at this dose (a single baby aspirin). Unfortunately, platelets have several activation pathways that bypass the inhibitory effect of aspirin. This is why aspirin, while its effectiveness is established for many clinical conditions, does not help everyone who takes it (3). It should be noted that platelets lack significant inducible COX-2 activity, and selective COX-2 inhibitors have *no* effect on platelet function.

Aspirin is indicated for conditions related to coronary artery disease (unstable angina, acute myocardial infarction with or without thrombolysis, and secondary prevention), coronary revascularization procedures (before angioplasty and after bypass grafting), carotid artery disease (transient ischemic attacks and secondary prevention), and peripheral artery disease (when used with dipyridamole). Although there are data that aspirin prevents a first heart attack, presently the American Heart Association does not recommend it (4). The U.S. Preventive Medicine Task Force recommends that "low dose aspirin therapy be considered for men age 40 and over who are at significantly increased risk of myocardial infarction and who lack contraindications to the drug." Caution is in order because of the risk of bleeding associated with aspirin therapy: about 5% for minor and about 1% for major bleeding. In the U.S. Physicians Health study of 22,000 male physicians receiving 325 mg of aspirin (or placebo) every other day, hemorrhagic stroke was observed in 0.2% of the aspirin group versus 0.1% of the placebo group (not statistically significant), but gastrointestinal bleeding requiring transfusions was significantly increased by aspirin (0.5% versus 0.3% in the placebo group). As a single agent, aspirin may be useful for nonvalvular atrial fibrillation in patients who cannot tolerate warfarin, but it is not useful in DVT prophylaxis or for the prevention of preeclampsia/eclampsia (5). More details are provided in Chapter 6.

Ticlopidine

Ticlopidine and clopidogrel are thienopyridine compounds that may be somewhat more potent platelet inhibitors than aspirin (6). Both are inactive in vitro, and both are converted to as yet undiscovered active metabolites by the liver. Their mechanism of action is uncertain, but appears to involve a receptor-level blockade of adenosine diphosphate (ADP) binding to platelets. Both require several days of treatment before platelet inhibition occurs, and their maximal effect is not seen for about 1 week after beginning the medication.

When aspirin and ticlopidine are used together following stenting, ADP-induced aggregation is inhibited within 2 days. When used for periods longer than 1 month, ticlopidine is associated with about a 2.5% incidence of neutropenia (with approximately 1% of patients whose neutrophil count falls below 500/µL), and a surprising number of cases of thrombotic thrombocytopenic purpura (TTP) (7). Equally surprising is the relatively small bleeding risk associated with ticlopidine (5% to 10% have minor bleeding and less than 1% have major bleeding, rates comparable to those associated with aspirin). Other side effects of both ticlopidine and clopidogrel are rashes, nausea, diarrhea, and possibly elevations of serum cholesterol.

Ticlopidine (250 mg, orally, twice a day) is currently indicated for use in the secondary prevention of stroke and transient ischemic attack, and for preventing coronary artery reocclusion after stent placement (250 mg, orally, twice a day for 1 month, given with aspirin). It appears also useful for decreasing the morbidity associated with peripheral artery disease and possibly decreasing the morbidity and mortality in patients with unstable angina and myocardial infarction.

Clopidogrel

Clopidogrel is structurally related to ticlopidine, with a similar mechanism of action but a toxicity profile that is muted. Neutropenia occurs very rarely (<1%) and TTP is an even rarer side effect (see Chapter 12). Clopidogrel (75 mg, orally, every day) has been FDA-approved for the reduction of ischemic events in patients who have had recent myocardial infarction, stroke, or peripheral artery disease, based on a study showing its superiority to aspirin (8).

Abciximab

Abciximab (ReoPro, Centocor) is a chimeric human-mouse Fab immunoglobulin fragment that binds to platelet GpIIb-IIIa and inhibits platelet cohesive interactions with fibrinogen and/or vWF. It is the prototypical inhibitor of the third phase of platelet responses, the final common pathway of platelet aggregation. As such, it presents a mechanism of action and therapeutic index that is similar to the two other structurally unique and commercially available GpIIb-IIIa inhibitors, eptifibatide and tirofiban.

The use of abciximab is optimized by bolus injection (0.25 mg/kg) followed by a continuous infusion of 0.125 µg/kg/min (max 10 µg/min) for 12 hours. This program is approved for use with angioplasty, where abciximab improves all measurable outcomes, including long-term survival. The primary toxicity is bleeding, which occurs in about 10% of patients receiving this dosing of the GpIIb-IIIa antagonist (9). Intracranial bleeding and death due to bleeding are extremely rare (0.3% and 0.09%, respectively). This occurs within the context of a patient simultaneously receiving aspirin and heparin. Attenuating the dose of heparin, early percutaneous sheath removal, and fastidious attention to the puncture site may reduce bleeding complications. Another rare side effect is thrombocytopenia, which, when defined by a fall in the platelet count to less than 50,000/µL, occurs in about 1% of patients. The bleeding complications of

Table 7.1   Contraindications to the use of parenteral GpIIb-IIIa antagonists

Active bleeding or a history of bleeding, including genitourinary or
    gastrointestinal bleeding, within 30 days
Blood pressure >200/110
Major surgery within 6 weeks
Nonhemorrhagic stroke within 30 days
Any history of hemorrhagic stroke
Pregnancy
Renal failure
Receipt of a thrombolytic agent within 24 hours

abciximab have forced the development of a long list of contraindications to its use (as well as the use of eptifibatide and tirofiban) (Table 7.1). It costs up to $1000 per course of treatment.

Tirofiban

Tirofiban (Aggrastat, Merck) is a non-peptide antagonist of the platelet GpIIb-IIIa receptor that binds to it with a higher affinity than its endogenous ligands fibrinogen and vWF. It is FDA-approved for use in unstable angina. It is administered as a bolus of 0.4 µg/kg followed by an infusion of 0.1 µg/kg/min for a minimum of 48 hours, and it works best when given with full-dose heparin and aspirin. Its toxicity profile is improved in comparison with abciximab (10). It costs about $500 to $1000 per course of treatment.

Eptifibatide

Eptifibatide (Integrilin, COR Therapeutics) is the most recently approved GpIIb-IIIa inhibitor. It is a cyclic peptide blocker of platelet aggregation, which has been given fairly broad indications for use: "acute coronary syndromes, including percutaneous coronary interventions." It is also administered as a bolus (180 µg/kg) followed by infusion (2 µg/kg/min) until the patient is discharged from the hospital or for 72 hours, whichever occurs first. It is also administered with heparin and aspirin, although the recommended dose of heparin targets an aPTT of 50 to 70 rather than two times control. It is associated with bleeding and thrombocytopenia, although to a lesser degree than abciximab (11,12). It costs a little more than $1000 per course of treatment.

Annotated Bibliography

1. Schafer AI. Antiplatelet therapy. Am J Med 1996;101:199–209.
    This is a comprehensive review of the molecular pharmacology of antiplatelet

drugs. It includes several figures that may help to elucidate mechanisms of action, as well as provide key understanding as to the shortcomings of currently available agents.

2. FitzGerald GA, Oates JA, Hawiger J, et al. Endogenous biosynthesis of prostacyclin and thromboxane and platelet function during chronic administration of aspirin in man. J Clin Invest 1983;71:676–688.

By measuring urinary metabolites of platelet thromboxane and vessel wall prostacyclin, these investigators provide strong clinical evidence that the therapeutic index of ingested aspirin is maximized by doses equivalent to or less than a single baby aspirin every day. When volunteers took 80 mg of aspirin per day for 7 days, thromboxane levels were decreased by 90%, while prostacyclin levels were reduced by 50%.

3. Roth GJ, Calverley DC. Aspirin, platelets, and thrombosis: theory and practice. Blood 1994;83:885–898.

A wonderfully well-written and informative review of basic and clinical information from the perspective of GJ Roth, a physician and scientist who discovered aspirin's mechanism of action.

4. Hennekens CH, Dyken ML, Fuster V. Aspirin as a therapeutic agent in cardiovascular disease: a statement for healthcare professionals from the American Heart Association. Circulation 1997;96:2751–2753.

This presents a brief practice guideline.

5. Caritis S, Sibai B, Hauth J, et al. Low-dose aspirin to prevent preeclampsia in women at high risk. New Engl J Med 1998;338:701–705.

This was a double-blind, randomized, placebo-controlled trial examining four groups of pregnant women at high risk for preeclampsia, including 471 women with pregestational insulin-treated diabetes mellitus, 774 women with chronic hypertension, 688 women with multifetal gestations, and 606 women who had preeclampsia during a previous pregnancy. The women were enrolled between gestational weeks 13 and 26 and received either 60 mg of aspirin or placebo daily. Outcome data were obtained on all but 36 of the 2539 women who entered the study. The incidence of preeclampsia was similar in the 1254 women in the aspirin group and the 1249 women in the placebo group (aspirin, 18%; placebo, 20%). The incidences in the aspirin and placebo groups for each of the four high-risk categories were also similar: for women with pregestational diabetes mellitus, the incidence was 18% percent in the aspirin group and 22% in the placebo group; for women with chronic hypertension, 26% and 25%; for those with multifetal gestations, 12% and 16%; and for those with preeclampsia during a previous pregnancy, 17% and 19%. The incidences of perinatal death, preterm birth, and infants small for gestational age were similar in the aspirin and placebo groups.

6. Sharis PJ, Cannon CP, Loscalzo J. The antiplatelet effects of ticlopidine and clopidogrel. Ann Intern Med 1998;129:394–405.

A thorough review of the biology and pharmacology of ticlopidine and clopidogrel. For those of you interested in the precise purinergic receptor acted upon by these agents, see *Nature* 2001; Vol 409; pages 202–206.

7. Bennett CL, Weinberg PD, Rozenberg-Ben-Dror K, et al. Thrombotic Thrombocytopenic purpura associated with ticlopidine. A review of 60 cases. Ann Inter Med 1998;128:541–544.

Ticlopidine is associated with the development of TTP, even when it is prescribed for only 1 month for patients with coronary artery stents. The prevalence of this complication is not known, but the risk should be discussed with patients and platelet counts monitored. The longest interval between beginning ticlopidine and the onset of TTP was 16 weeks; the shortest was 1 week.

8. CAPRIE Steering Committee. A randomised, blinded trial of clopidogrel versus aspirin in patients at risk of ischaemic events (CAPRIE). Lancet 1996;348:1329–1339.

CAPRIE was a randomised, blinded, international trial designed to assess the relative efficacy of clopidogrel (75 mg once daily) and aspirin (325 mg once daily) in reducing the risk of a composite outcome cluster of ischemic stroke, myocardial infarction, or vascular death. The population examined was followed for 1 to 3 years and was comprised of subgroups of patients with atherosclerotic vascular disease manifested as either recent ischemic stroke, recent myocardial infarction, or symptomatic peripheral arterial disease. 19,185 patients, with more than 6300 in each of the clinical subgroups, were recruited over 3 years, with a mean follow-up of 1.91 years. There were 1960 new events. Clopidogrel-treated persons had an annual 5.32% risk of ischaemic stroke, myocardial infarction, or vascular death compared with 5.83% with aspirin. These rates reflect a small but statistically significant ($P = 0.043$) relative-risk reduction of 8.7% in favor of clopidogrel. There were no major differences in terms of safety.

9. Aguirre FV, Topol EJ, Ferguson JJ, et al. Bleeding complications with the chimeric antibody to platelet glycoprotein IIb/IIIa integrin in patients undergoing percutaneous coronary intervention. EPIC Investigators. Circulation 1995;91:2882–2890.

Bleeding complications were two to three times more frequent in patients receiving abciximab than in those receiving placebo, but most were transient and well tolerated. Risk-factor analysis and modification of concomitant antithrombotic and antiplatelet treatment strategies may aid in reducing bleeding complications during percutaneous coronary revascularization.

10. PRISM Study Group. Inhibition of the platelet glycoprotein IIb/IIIa receptor with tirofiban in unstable angina and non-Q-wave myocardial infarction. New Engl J Med 1998;338:1488–1504.

Tirofiban, aspirin, plus heparin was superior to aspirin plus heparin in this phase 3 study of 1915 patients. The improvements in rates of death, myocardial infarction, and refractory ischemia persisted for up to 6 months after treatment. Major bleeding (Hgb fall of 4 grams/dL, 2 or more units of red blood cells transfused, need for corrective surgery, and/or intracranial or retroperitoneal bleeding) occurred in 4% of the tirofiban group and 3% of the control group.

11. The PURSUIT Trial Investigators. Inhibition of platelet glycoprotein IIb/IIIa with eptifibatide in patients with acute coronary syndromes. New Engl J Med 1998;339:436–443.

A large study of almost 11,000 patients with transient ST-segment elevation and/or elevations of creatinine kinase MB isoenzymes. Eptifibatide (Integrilin) benefited almost all patient groups, including those receiving percutaneous interventions (PTCA and stenting). The benefit was measured as the incidence of death or nonfatal myocardial infarction at 30 days out from the ischemic event: 14.2% in the eptifibatide/heparin/aspirin group versus 15.7% in the heparin/aspirin-alone group. Bleeding was increased in the eptifibatide group, particularly mild bleeding, but the incidence of operative bleeding (CABG) and intracranial hemorrhage was no different between the two groups.

12. Lefkovits J, Plow EF, Topol EJ. Platelet glycoprotein IIb/IIIa receptors in cardiovascular medicine. New Engl J Med 1995;332:1553–1559.

A broad review of the pathophysiology and treatment of platelet-dependent thrombosis from a cardiologist's point of view. Included are some of the chemical structures of these inhibitors, including tirofiban.

8

Thrombolytic Therapy

Thrombolytic therapy can be used for acute myocardial infarction (MI), pulmonary embolism (PE), deep venous thrombosis (DVT), ischemic stroke, and for clearing catheters and cannulae. It works by dissolving the fibrin clot, as well as the fibrinogen and vWF nexus that pulls platelets together into a thrombus. The life span of a thrombus normally includes physiological thrombolysis mediated primarily by plasmin generated from plasma plasminogen by tissue plasminogen activator released by the vessel wall (see Fig. 1.4). This occurs continually within our vascular tree to prevent thrombosis with normal "wear and tear," and it has been shown to occur days to weeks after an acute thrombosis of either arteries or veins. Pharmacological fibrinolysis is employed to restore flow to protect ischemic tissues from progressive damage (as in MI, stroke, and PE) or to enhance vessel lumen remodeling that favors a return to normal function (DVT).

To achieve these goals, thrombolytic therapy must be administered within a short period after the onset of the thrombosis. The usefulness of thrombolysis is limited to a time frame that changes with the site of thrombus formation: within 3 hours of a stroke, within 6 hours of an MI (there may be an benefit up to 24 hours), and as soon as the diagnosis of DVT or PE is established (although there can be therapeutic benefits up to 7 days after the onset of venous thromboembolism). The indications for thrombolytic therapy are fairly narrow because its therapeutic index is precipitously narrow: bleeding is a very serious side effect. For this reason, thrombolytic therapy must be used judiciously, with careful consideration of contraindications that might apply for each patient. It is also for this reason that thrombolytic therapy has become mainstream primarily only for acute MI, even though both streptokinase and urokinase have been approved by the Food and Drug Administration for use in treating PE for over two decades.

The Risk-Benefit Ratio of Thrombolytic Therapy

It is reasonable to approach the use of thrombolytics for acute MI by focusing on their benefits, and then considering risk. This is because of their clear-cut effect on improving mortality (see Chapter 6) and their large-scale routine use in this setting (50% of all patients with acute MI). It is just as reasonable to focus on risk of thrombolytic therapy when considering its use for patients with venous thromboembolism. This is because there are no data that mortality is improved when thrombolytics are administered to patients with DVT or PE. There is a consensus, however, that thrombolytics should be used routinely in patients with "massive" PE, defined as a PE associated with threatened or overt cardiovascular collapse, although even in this setting their impact on survival is not clear-cut.

The obvious risk of thrombolytic therapy is bleeding, and the most serious hemorrhagic side effect that must be confronted when considering its use is fatal intracranial bleeding. When a conventional dosage of tissue plasminogen activator (tPA) is used for acute MI (see Chapter 6), patients will bleed into their head and die: of 71,073 patients so treated, 673 (0.95%) had intracranial bleeding (1). Of these patients, 331 (53%) died and 158 (25%) had residual neurological deficits. Despite this, the overall benefit of tPA is at least a 1% improvement in mortality, and its therapeutic index is clearly favorable. Perhaps the primary goal of large-scale clinical research in this area is to identify new agents, or new dose schedules for old agents, that provide incremental improvements in the therapeutic index for using thrombolytic agents in acute MI.

The individual clinician can improve the therapeutic index of thrombolytic agents by considering all of the standard contraindications: active internal bleeding, a history of stroke, intracranial or intraspinal surgery within 2 months, recent trauma including cardiopulmonary resuscitation, intracranial neoplasm/arteriovenous malformations/aneurysms, a bleeding diathesis, and severe uncontrolled hypertension. In addition, careful monitoring of dosing (for example, stay below a 1.5 mg/kg total tPA dose and watch out for overdosing the patients who have lower body weights) should become a routine part of all clinicians' approaches to their patients receiving thrombolytic therapy. Finally, but perhaps most importantly, morbidity can be reduced by vigilant attention to sites of vascular invasion, particularly arterial punctures, including aggressive and durable compression of puncture sites.

There is currently no particularly useful way to monitor thrombolytic therapy specifically, although the aPTT and thrombin time are increased as a consequence of thrombolytic therapy. The *activated clotting time* (ACT) is a simple method, applicable at the bedside, that is frequently used to monitor patients receiving tPA plus heparin for MI. Blood is drawn into tubes containing kaolin, and the time to gelation is measured. The ACT, although not sensitive in a predictable way to tPA, helps guide heparin dosing in this situation: to minimize hemorrhagic complications, heparin doses should be decreased when the ACT is over 200 seconds.

Thrombolytic Agents Available in the United States

Thrombolysis for venous thromboembolic disorders, myocardial infarction, and stroke was described previously in Chapters 4 and 6. The following summary provides indications and practical guidelines for using each of the thrombolytic agents available for use by physicians in the United States.

Streptokinase

In MI, a single dose of 1,500,000 IU is infused over 1 hour. In PE, DVT, and arterial thromboembolism, 250,000 IU is infused over the first 30 minutes. This is followed by 100,000 IU per hour for 24 hours (PE), 72 hours (DVT), or 24 to 72 hours (arterial occlusion). The half-life of streptokinase is about 30 minutes. Obstructed atrioventricular cannulae are cleared by 250,000 IU clamped inside the cannula for 2 hours. Streptokinase causes allergic reactions—including symptoms of fever, rash, rigor, and/or bronchospasm—in about 5% of those who receive it. Hypotension is a common side effect. Hypotension requiring pressor therapy usually develops within the first hour of treatment and affects at least 5% of all those who receive streptokinase. Anaphylaxis is uncommon, with about 1 out of 1000 patients developing this side effect. Streptokinase induces the production of neutralizing antibodies within just a few days of its infusion, and these antibodies last for several years. For this reason, no patients should receive thrombolytic therapy with streptokinase for at least 1 year following its initial use. At that time, if you are considering using it, make sure that antibody titers are low. If there is any concern about delivering the effective dose of streptokinase, use another thrombolytic agent.

Tissue Plasminogen Activator (tPA)

A standard dosing regimen in acute MI is presented in Chapter 6. An alternative dosing strategy is referred to as "accelerated" tPA. For patients weighing over 67 kg, it is administered as follows: 100 mg over 15 minutes, followed by 50 mg over 30 minutes, followed by 35 over 60 minutes. For patients weighing less than 67 kg, it is given differently: 15 mg over 10 minutes, followed by 0.75 mg/kg over 30 minutes, followed by 0.5 mg/kg over 60 minutes. For stroke patients who are able to receive it within 3 hours of the onset of symptoms, tPA is given at a dose of 0.9 mg/kg (maximum of 90 mg) infused over 60 minutes, with 10% of the dose given as an initial 1-minute bolus. For venous thromboembolism, including "massive PE," 100 mg is infused over 2 hours. The half-life of tPA is only a few minutes. Therefore, in all cases except stroke, the optimal outcome is achieved when heparin anticoagulation is started during or shortly after the tPA infusion is completed. tPA does not commonly cause allergic symptoms, but profound hypotension develops in about 4% of treated patients.

Anisoylated Plasminogen–SK Complex (APSAC)

Anisoylated plasminogen-SK complex (APSAC) is a chemically engineered drug in which streptokinase is noncovalently bonded to plasminogen. The fibrin recognition site of plasminogen remains available, but the active catalytic site of plasminogen is "blocked" by the addition of a ringed anisoyl group. Following infusion, the plasminogen targets the complex to solid phase fibrin, while the blocking group is slowly removed by deacetylases present in plasma, thus permitting the SK to activate it. This results in some relative specificity for fibrin clots and a prolonged therapeutic half-life of about 90 minutes. APSAC is approved for use only in MI. For this indication, 30 units are infused over 2 to 5 minutes as soon as possible after the onset of symptoms and then full-dose heparin is started. APSAC cannot be given to patients who have been recently given streptokinase, and should not be given to persons who have suffered allergic reactions to streptokinase. The incidence of allergic reactions, hypotension, and anaphylaxis in response to APSAC is similar to the incidence with streptokinase.

Reteplase (rPA)

Reteplase (rPA) is a genetically engineered nonglycosylated mutant of tPA containing only the second kringle and catalytic domains. It has a very prolonged half-life in comparison to tPA (58 versus 3 minutes). It is indicated for the treatment of acute MI: it is given as a 10 mg bolus over 2 minutes, followed by a second 10 mg bolus 30 minutes after the first. Other than bleeding, side effects are uncommon. Reteplase may someday be deemed safe enough to be administered outside of the hospital by emergency personnel responding to persons with acute MI.

Urokinase

For pulmonary embolism, 4400 IU/kg of urokinase is infused over 10 minutes, followed by 4400 IU/kg/hour for 12 hours. A heparin infusion is started without a loading dose when the thrombin time is less than 2 times normal (about 3 to 4 hours after urokinase, which has a half-life of about 30 minutes, has been stopped). Urokinase is approved only for intracoronary artery thrombolysis, where it is used infrequently and only by skilled subspecialists. Urokinase, because it is a human product, almost never causes allergic side effects.

Management of Bleeding

For patients receiving thrombolytic therapy, the short half-life of the agents simplifies the clinicians' response to any bleeding that develops: the first and often the only step needed is to stop the infusion. All heparin and anti-platelet GpIIb-IIIa infusions should be stopped. Heparin reversal with protamine should be considered if a subcutaneous injection was the route of administration. When possible, pressure should be applied to the site of bleeding. Patients with persistently elevated thrombin times off heparin should have the plasma fibrinogen level measured; if the level is less than 100 mg/dL, cryoprecipitate should be given. There are no specific antidotes to thrombolytic agents. ε Aminocaproic acid and tranexamic acid inhibit plasmin directly, and could be used in patients who are exsanguinating from thrombolytic therapy. Aprotinin is a much more potent inhibitor of plasmin, but it is not approved for use in this setting. All antiplasmin agents are associated with a risk of thrombosis and disseminated intravascular coagulation (DIC), so they should be avoided in patients with hematuria or liver disease. Other than reversing all iatrogenic hemostatic defects, there are no specific interventions currently available that favorably affect the natural history of intracranial bleeding associated with thrombolytic therapy.

Annotated Bibliography

1. Gurwitz JH, Gore JM, Goldberg RJ, et al. Risk of intracranial hemorrhage after tissue plasminogen activator treatments for acute myocardial infarction. Ann Intern Med 1989;129:597–604.

   Intracranial hemorrhage occurs in almost 1% of patients who receive tPA for MI. Appropriate drug dosing and avoidance of patients with risk factors, particularly those with a history of stroke, will decrease the incidence of intracranial hemorrhage in these patients.

2. Sane DC, Califf RM, Topol EJ, et al. Bleeding during thrombolytic therapy for acute myocardial infarction: mechanisms and management. Ann Intern Med 1989;111:1010–1022.

   A thorough review of the subject, including some treatment algorithms that have not become outdated.

9

Lupus Anticoagulants, Antiphospholipid Antibodies, and the Antiphospholipid Syndrome

Lupus anticoagulants, antiphospholipid antibodies, and the antiphospholipid syndrome are subjects usually lumped together. This is a good thing because one cannot understand one without understanding the others. But it is bad because it can confuse the practitioner—who then is at risk for overinterpreting or underinterpreting their clinical significance. Therefore, some definitions are needed. *Lupus anticoagulants* are autoantibodies that affect phospholipid-dependent coagulation tests (Fig. 9.1). Almost all lupus anticoagulants are *antiphospholipid antibodies* (APAs), but not all APAs are lupus anticoagulants (only about 1/4 [1–2]). APAs are identified by their reactivity with a solid phospholipid surface that is most commonly cardiolipin (Fig. 9.2). The *antiphospholipid syndrome* is defined as the association of an APA (with or without a lupus anticoagulant) with venous thromboembolic disease, arterial thrombosis, recurrent second trimester miscarriage, and/or thrombocytopenia. In persons who suffer from these problems, the presence of an APA defines a clinically relevant entity that must be treated, and it is treated with warfarin (except in pregnancy) targeted to an internationalized normalized ratio (INR) that is higher than usual (aim for an INR of 3.0–3.5).

On the other end of the spectrum are the clinically irrelevant lupus anticoagulants and/or APAs that develop in aging patients, patients infected with HIV or syphilis, and patients treated with certain medications. These phenomena should be ignored. Some practical issues can be teased out of this confusing nomenclature to create the following generalizations:

1. Lupus anticoagulants are more likely to be clinically relevant.
2. No lupus anticoagulant or APA needs to be treated preemptively.

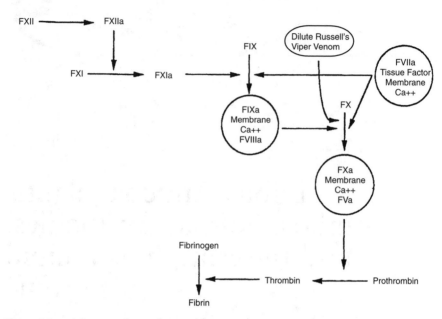

Figure 9.1. A lupus anticoagulant prolongs an aPTT or, less commonly, a PT, because it interferes with the phospholipid-dependent coagulation reactions (circled). A dilute Russell's viper venom time is a more sensitive assay because it is a less potent direct activator of factor X; a less avid or lower titer antibody to phospholipid is therefore more likely to affect this route of activation of the "prothrombinase" complex. (Reproduced by permission from Galli M, Barbui T. Antiprothrombin antibodies: detection and clinical significance in the antiphospholipid syndrome. Blood 1999;93:2149–2157.)

3. *Both* lupus anticoagulants and an APA should be looked for in two common diseases in younger individuals with no obvious risk factors for getting them: venous thromboembolism and stroke.

4. An APA should be looked for in women with recurrent second trimester miscarriage or fetal death of unknown etiology.

5. *Both* lupus anticoagulants and APAs must be looked for at least twice with a 3-month interval between tests. The majority of these phenomena are ephemeral (80% to 90% disappear after 1 year), but a persistent or increasing APA is more likely associated with clinically relevant events (3).

Lupus Anticoagulant

Four criteria must be satisfied to establish the presence of a lupus anticoagulant (4):

1. A phospholipid-dependent coagulation test is prolonged.

2. There is no correction of the abnormal test with mixing.

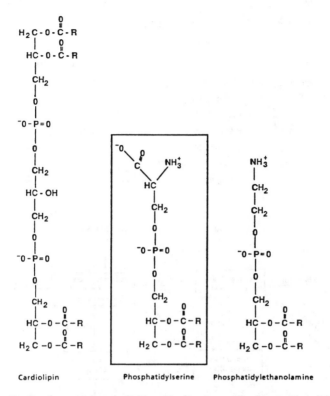

Cardiolipin   Phosphatidylserine   Phosphatidylethanolamine

Figure 9.2. Testing for antiphospholipid antibodies is usually done with solid-phase phospholipid, such as cardiolipin or phosphatidylserine. These anionic phospholipids bind to β_2-glycoprotein 1, which is the most common target of an APA. The APA recognizes the lipid/protein complex. A sensitive test for APAs uses phosphatidylethanolamine concentrated in an aqueous solution so that it forms a barrel-like "hexagonal" phase structure with its polar (charged) phosphodiester-linked head group directed out and its nonpolar (hydrophobic) acyl groups pointing in. (Reproduced with permission from Loscalzo J, Schafer AI, eds. Thrombosis and hemorrhage. 2nd ed. Philadelphia: Lippincott Williams & Wilkins, 1998. Copyright © 1998, Lippincott Williams & Wilkins Co.)

3. The addition of phospholipid corrects the abnormal test.

4. A specific factor inhibitor or other coagulopathy is ruled out.

None of the laboratory testing criteria are standardized. Table 9.1 lists in rank order those tests that are used commonly to satisfy these criteria. Figure 9.3 provides an algorithm for using several of these tests (4). Physicians should confirm with the clinical laboratory the tests upon which the report of a "positive lupus anticoagulant" is based.

Lupus anticoagulants are found most commonly associated with the disease lupus (about 7% of patients in one study [1–2]), but they are also found associated with other autoimmune disorders and often arise de novo. The "lupus

Table 9.1   Tests to establish the presence of a lupus anticoagulant

	TEST	SENSITIVITY
Screening	aPTT	Good
	Kaolin clotting time	Better
	Dilute RVVT	Better
Mixing	Plasma 1:1	Very good (~85%)
	With incubation	Excellent (~100%)
Confirmatory	Platelet neutralization	Excellent
	Hexagonal phase phospholipid	Excellent

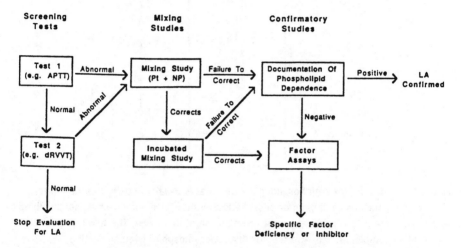

Figure 9.3.   A flow chart for an approach to the diagnosis of a lupus anticoagulant (LA) is illustrated. The evaluation begins with one or more screen assays. At least two screening assays, based on different properties, should be performed before the possibility of an LA is eliminated. These screening tests can be performed concurrently or sequentially, depending on the operation of the testing laboratory. If either of the screening tests is abnormal, mixing studies would be performed to determine if an inhibitor is present. If the initial mixing study shows correction of the abnormal clotting time, then an assay for time-dependent inhibition should be performed. If the mixing studies indicate the presence of a circulating inhibitor, then LA confirmatory studies should be performed that examines the capacity of excess phospholipid (derived from platelets or hexagonal phase phosphatidylethanolamine) to absorb and "neutralize" the LA. Such assays should be based on the test system giving the abnormal screen assay. Factor assays may be used when the mixing studies show correction, suggesting a factor deficiency, when the LA confirmatory studies are negative or when a specific factor inhibitor is suspected. (Reproduced by permission from Brandt JT, Triplett DA, Alving B, Scharrer I. Criteria for the diagnosis of lupus anticoagulants: an update. On behalf of the Subcommittee on Lupus Anticoagulant/Antiphospholipid Antibody of the Scientific and Standardisation Committee of the ISTH. Thromb Haemost 1995;74:1185–1190.)

Table 9.2 **Clinically trivial lupus anticoagulants**

Children

Elderly

HIV/AIDS

Infections (syphilis, Lyme disease, adenovirus, rubella, varicella,
tuberculosis)

Medication (procainamide, INH, chlorpromazine, methyldopa, hydralazine,
quinidine)

anticoagulant" does not anticoagulate blood. On the contrary, in both lupus-associated and de novo cases, there is a 15% to 20% lifetime risk that the person will suffer a venous thrombosis and a 10% to 15% risk that the person will suffer an arterial thrombosis. Thus, the lupus anticoagulant is a common cause of the *hypercoagulable state*. In fact, 15% to 20% of all hypercoagulable cases are caused by the lupus anticoagulant or an APA (see Chapter 10). It only rarely causes bleeding (see below). When the lupus anticoagulant is discovered incidentally in children, in the elderly, or as secondary to a nonconnective tissue disorder or a medication (Table 9.2), it is clinically trivial in almost 100% of individuals.

Antiphospholipid Antibody

An antiphospholipid antibody is an IgG or IgM autoantibody that binds to proteins that form a complex with anionic phospholipids. In some (perhaps most) cases, an APA is actually directed to the protein alone, although under in vivo and most in vitro conditions (i.e., ELISA analyses in which the plate is blocked with fetal serum) the components of the protein/phospholipid complex are inseparable. There is little correlation between the type or titer of the antibody and the presence or magnitude of a lupus anticoagulant, although there may be a correlation between type and titer of APA and the risk of thrombosis or spontaneous abortion (5). Some of the phospholipid-binding proteins recognized by an APA are, in descending order of importance, β_2-glycoprotein I (β2-GPI), prothrombin, annexin V, activated protein C, and protein S. The major phospholipid that these proteins interact with in vivo is probably phosphatidylserine (PS), but in vitro antiphospholipid antibodies recognize these proteins attached to any anionic phospholipid, including phosphatidylethanolamine, cardiolipin, or phosphatidylserine (6). The most commonly used assay, and therefore the most commonly encountered APA, is an anticardiolipin antibody.

Because some protein/phospholipid complexes recognized by antiphospholipid antibodies regulate coagulation reactions, antiphospholipid antibodies can sometimes affect hemostasis and thrombosis (see Fig. 9.1). When they affect a phospholipid-dependent coagulation reaction, APAs are designated as *lupus anticoagulants*. Whereas lupus anticoagulants are found in about 7% to 40%

of patients with lupus, APAs are found in 25% to 60%, attesting to the relative overlap among these two laboratory tests and the greater sensitivity of the direct APA assay in comparison to the lupus anticoagulant assays. Like a lupus anticoagulant, the presence of an APA in someone with lupus or a related disease is associated with a risk for venous thrombosis, arterial thrombosis (particularly stroke), or recurrent spontaneous abortion. In addition, several less frequent clinical associations have been reported, including thrombocytopenia, cardiac valvular abnormalities, livedo reticularis, and optic nerve ischemia. When these thrombotic phenomena occur in a patient without a connective tissue disorder, that person suffers from the *primary antiphospholipid antibody syndrome*. Like the lupus anticoagulant, an APA is clinically insignificant when it is discovered incidentally in the conditions listed in Table 9.2.

Pathophysiology

The mechanisms by which APAs lead to thrombosis remain speculative. When one considers the protein targets of APAs, however, certain reasonable hypotheses about the pathophysiology of venous thrombosis emerge. β_2-Glycoprotein 1 circulates in plasma at a concentration of $200\,\mu g/mL$. Its physiological role is uncertain, but its avidity for anionic phospholipids raises the possibility that it serves as a natural anticoagulant by blocking coagulation factor assembly on the surface of stimulated platelets, which "flip" phosphatidylserine (PS) from the inner to outer plasma membrane after activation. Thus, an APA directed against β_2-glycoprotein 1 could theoretically eliminate this normal homeostatic antithrombotic mechanism by increasing the clearance of β_2-glycoprotein 1 or decreasing its avidity for the surface of activated platelets. An APA directed against this protein could also theoretically bind to the β_2-glycoprotein 1/PS complex on activated platelets, increasing their uptake by splenic macrophages and causing an immune-type thrombocytopenia, which is present in about 20% of patients with the primary APA syndrome (7).

When an APA is directed against activated protein C (APC) or its cofactor protein S, hypercoagulability is easy to explain: these patients have an acquired APC or protein S deficiency. Similarly, because annexin V is a natural anticoagulant that is proven to function as an inhibitor of phospholipid-dependent coagulation factor assembly and activation, an APA directed specifically at annexin V that inhibits its activity would cause hypercoagulability. A conundrum that runs through these speculations about the mechanism of APA's hypercoagulable effect, however, is that each of the molecules that have been described primarily regulates venous (coagulation factor induced) thrombosis, without any obvious effect on platelet-dependent arterial thrombosis. Although there are reports of APAs that activate platelets, this effect is not universal and we are left with even greater uncertainty about how an APA might cause stroke or myocardial infarction.

Very rarely, a patient acquires clinically significant hypoprothrombinemia because of an APA that binds to prothrombin (8). These occur spontaneously, and can also develop in patients with connective tissue disorders and viral infections. A lupus anticoagulant and/or APA secondary to a pediatric viral syndrome that results in bleeding from prothrombin deficiency is the only predictable (albeit uncommon) exception to the observation that infection-associated lupus anticoagulants or APAs are clinically trivial (see Table 9.2).

Clinical Complications

The clinical manifestations of a pathological APA are mainly thrombosis and second trimester fetal loss. The thrombi develop in both venous and arterial circuits; a recent retrospective review of 360 persons with APA showed an equal number of venous and arterial thrombosis, 17 each (3). The most common site of venous thrombosis in this study is the legs (9 of 17 patients in one study), and the most common site of arterial thrombosis is the cerebral circulation (16 of 17 patient had stroke or transient ischemic attack in that study). Fetal death or spontaneous abortions typically occur in the second trimester as a consequence of placental insufficiency. In the study referred to above, 11 of 28 pregnancies among women were abortive, with 9 of 16 occurring in women who had had previous miscarriages or thromboses, and only 2 of 12 developing without any history of an antecedent complication. As stated above, the antiphospholipid syndrome is defined by more than one (two or more) episodes of fetal death. It is, nonetheless, reasonable to test for an APA in all women after a single unexplained second trimester miscarriage, although the benefit of treatment after a *single* fetal loss is not established. On the other hand, there is no reason to measure an APA in primiparous women or multiparous women who have suffered a first trimester miscarriage, unless there has been recurrent spontaneous first trimester abortions without any cause established.

A less dangerous manifestation of both primary and secondary APA syndromes is livedo reticularis. Both primary and secondary APA syndromes are also associated with heart valve abnormalities, particularly left-sided vegetations that cause insufficiency (9). Patients with the primary APA syndrome may also suffer vascular headaches and visual symptoms besides amaurosis fugax. About 20% of patients have mild thrombocytopenia, which may increase the risk of bleeding during anticoagulant therapy.

Management

Secondary APL

1. Treat the underlying condition.
2. Target the warfarin to an INR of 3.0–3.5.
3. Monitor the APL: if it declines or disappears, stop the warfarin.

Primary APL

1. Target the warfarin to an INR of 3.0–3.5.
2. Monitor the APL: if it declines or disappears, stop the warfarin.

APL patient who has suffered at least two second trimester miscarriages

1. Administer acetylsalicylic acid (ASA) 81 mg orally, once a day, while the patient is attempting to conceive and throughout the pregnancy.
2. Administer unfractionated heparin, 5000 U subcutaneously, twice a day; or enoxaparin, 30 mg subcutaneously, once a day, during the pregnancy and for 8 weeks postpartum.

Full anticoagulation with heparin is used to treat an acute thrombosis. Because a lupus anticoagulant can affect the aPTT, one must target an aPTT that is 1.5 to 2.0 times the baseline value. Where it is available, measuring factor X activity is a more precise way to control heparin anticoagulation. Similarly, a lupus anticoagulant can affect the baseline INR. Even when the baseline INR is normal, lupus anticoagulants tend to make the INR on warfarin less reliable, and activated factor X levels provide more precise monitoring (10).

Factor X is measured by a simple automated assay that involves its activation (by Russell's viper venom in recalcified serum) followed by spectrophotometric monitoring of its cleavage of a chromogenic substrate. It has not yet displaced routine monitoring with the aPTT and INR, but if the patient's thrombosis recurrence or bleeding complication rates exceed the norms, factor X levels should be checked, cross-referenced with controls and standards, and correlated with the INRs measured for your patient in the laboratory. As a rule of thumb, recurrence among patients with an INR over 3.0 should be about one or two per 100 patients per year; mild bleeding can be expected in about seven patients, and severe bleeding in about two patients per 100 patients treated per year (11–12).

Although aspirin is often used in conjunction with anticoagulant therapy, it contributes nothing to the benefits of warfarin targeted appropriately (or heparin in pregnant patients), and it probably increases the bleeding risk. Similarly, there is no benefit from using corticosteroids to treat the APA syndrome (unless there is an antiprothrombin antibody causing bleeding), although they need not be withheld in patients with the secondary APA syndrome among whom there may be another indication for their use.

Annotated Bibliography

1. Petri M, Rheinschmidt M, Whiting-O'Keefe Q, et al. The frequency of lupus anticoagulant in systemic lupus erythematosus. A study of sixty consecutive patients by activated partial thromboplastin time, Russell viper venom time, and anticardiolipin antibody level. Ann Intern Med 1987;106:524–531.

2. Love P, Santoro S. Antiphospholipid antibodies: anticardiolipin and the lupus anticoagulant systemic lupus erythematosus (SLE) and in non-SLE disorders. Prevalence and clinical significance. Ann Intern Med 1990;112:682–698.

These papers provide prevalence data for a population of SLE patients that serves as a good index of the sensitivity and clinical significance of lupus anticoagulants and antiphospholipid antibodies. Out of 60 patients described in Petri et al., 4 (about 7%) had an elevated aPTT, 4 (about 7%) had an elevated dilute RVVT (only one of whom also had an elevated aPTT), and 15 (25%) had an anticardiolipin antibody. Clinically significant thromboses occurred in 1 out of 4 of the patients with increased aPTT, in 4 out of 4 with increased dRVVT, and in 8 out of 15 with the APA. Love and Santoro offer a literature review that reports that 34% of lupus patients have a lupus anticoagulant and 44% have an APA. The bottom line? An APA test is the most sensitive measure (i.e., the best screening test when working up a patient for "hypercoagulability"), and a functional test is the best predictor of clinical risk. Because there is no predictable overlap, both measures should be used when evaluating a person for nonfamilial thrombophilia. These concepts apply also to patients being evaluated for the primary APA syndrome.

3. Finazzi G, Brancaccio V, Moia M, et al. Natural history and risk factors for thrombosis in 360 patients with antiphospholipid antibodies: a four year prospective study from the Italian registry. Am J Med 1996;100:530–536.

   This is a descriptive analysis of 326 patients with a lupus anticoagulant and 185 patients with an IgG to cardiolipin. The rate of thrombosis was less than 10% among patients with an APA titer under 40 U, about 10% among patients with a lupus anticoagulant, and 20% to 25% among patients with an APA titer of over 40 U. An antecedent thrombotic event, including miscarriage, was associated with a fivefold risk of thrombosis in a patient with any laboratory abnormality.

4. Brandt J, Triplett D, Alving B, Scharrer I. Criteria for the diagnosis of lupus anticoagulants: an update. On behalf of the Subcommittee on Lupus. Anticoagulant/Antiphospholipid Antibody of the Scientific and Standardization Committee of the ISTH. Thromb Haemost 1995;74:1185–1190.

   The International Society for Thrombosis and Haemostasis works vigorously to develop standards for clinical reagents, and to assist clinical facilities with their proper use and interpretation. This paper summarizes such useful information about lupus anticoagulants.

5. Lockshin MD. Pregnancy loss in the antiphospholipid syndrome. Thromb Haemost 1999;82:641–648.

   This is a comprehensive review by a clinical investigator who has worked in this field for over two decades. It provides many detailed criteria around which high-impact clinical decisions could be made, including subdividing pregnant women into various risk groups and offering a complete analysis of their treatment options, ultimately boiled down into focused recommendations.

6. Roubey R. Autoantibodies to phospholipid-binding plasma proteins: a new view of lupus anticoagulants and other "antiphospholipid" autoantibodies. Blood 1994;84:2854–2867.

Everything you might want to know about the specificity of the autoantibodies that compose the APAs is included in this study written with an eye toward pathophysiology. The investigators make a plea for studies to elucidate their causes. The information reviewed also can help one to understand laboratory testing for APAs.

7. Thiagaragan P, Shapiro S. Coagulation disorders. Lupus anticoagulants and antiphospholipid antibodies. Hematol Oncol Clin North Am 1998;12:1167–1192.

This is the most comprehensive and recent review about the subject of this chapter.

8. Galli M, Barbui T. Antiprothrombin antibodies: detection and clinical significance in the antiphospholipid syndrome. Blood 1999;93:2149–2157.

A comprehensive review of antiprothrombin antibodies. Their general prevalence is not known, but they cause bleeding and should be looked for in patients with an APA who bleed excessively without an established cause. In such a patient, corticosteroids are the treatment of choice. In asymptomatic patients with an antiprothrombin antibody, standard treatment for thrombosis should be given even though the risk for bleeding is probably increased. The antiprothrombin antibody can elevate baseline PTs and INRs, and may make it difficult to monitor warfarin anticoagulation.

9. Galve E, Ordi J, Barquinero J, et al. Valvular heart disease in the primary antiphospholipid syndrome. Ann Intern Med 1992;116:293–298.

A case-control study of 28 patients with the primary APA syndrome. Ten patients had left-sided valve involvement, including eight with mitral and/or aorta insufficiency murmurs. Regurgitation was severe in two, moderate in three, and mild in three patients. No right-sided lesions were discovered.

10. Moll S, Ortel T. Monitoring warfarin therapy in patients with lupus anticoagulants. Ann Intern Med 1997;127:177–185.

Common sense is validated: if a lupus anticoagulant affects the reliability of INR measurements, then INR measurements should be replaced by a reproducible test that is not artifactually altered by a lupus anticoagulant. The questions that a practitioner must ask are how often is the INR affected (at least 25%) and how adverse are the consequences (not known). Therefore, although it is a terribly important issue to consider when interpreting data about optimal anticoagulation in these patients (particularly data from ongoing clinical trials), it is premature to discard INR measurements for monitoring warfarin dosing for patients with an APA.

11. Rosove M, Brewer P. Antiphospholipid thrombosis: clinical course after the first thrombotic event in 70 patients. Ann Intern Med 1992;117:303–308.

12. Khamashta M, Cuadrado M, Mujic F, et al. The management of thrombosis in the antiphospholipid-antibody syndrome. N Engl J Med 1995;332:993–997.

These papers direct our current standard of care in the oral anticoagulant therapy of patients with thromboses related to lupus anticoagulants or APAs. Warfarin dosed to an INR of 3.0 or greater is this standard. Aspirin is not useful and can increase the risk of bleeding. When the INR is below 3.0 the risk of recurrent thrombosis increases nearly 20-fold from 1.3 in 100 to 23 in 100 persons per year. At the therapeutic INR, severe bleeding occurs in about 2.5 of 100 persons per year.

10

Hypercoagulable States

Persons who are at an increased risk for developing a pathological thrombosis are called *hypercoagulable* or are described as suffering from *thrombophilia*. Most hypercoagulable states are from an acquired condition superimposed on some genetic predisposition, and are often multifactorial in origin. In some cases a cause is never established, but most of the time one can identify the trigger and the genetic and/or acquired predisposing factors. This interplay between nature and nurture can, in some cases, predict the natural history for a patient who has suffered a first event, and an understanding of the natural history can sometimes be used to direct the appropriate therapeutic plan.

Please remember that thrombosis involves the venous system, the arterial system, or both, and that specific hypercoagulable states will similarly involve venous thromboembolism, myocardial infarction, stroke, or rarely all three diseases (Table 10.1).

Epidemiology

Venous thromboembolism (VTE) affects on average about 1 in 1000 people per year. Age-adjusted incidence rates range from 1 in 10,000 for young patients, to 1 in 100 for the elderly (see Table 10.1). Among those with a first VTE, one or more significant pathogenetic hypercoagulable factors will be identified in the majority of patients (see Table 10.1). The hunt for a genetic cause is high yield in those with a family history of VTE (70%), but of lesser yield in those without a family history.

Unfortunately, in most cases the prognostic or therapeutic significance of identifying a genetic abnormality is vague and only rarely will it direct a modification of the standard treatment program. In contrast, identification of certain acquired hypercoagulable conditions is followed by almost a knee-jerk reaction to optimize the treatment plan. Two examples of this are raising the target INR and considering life-long anticoagulation after identifying a lupus anticoagulant (see Chapter 9), or modifying a woman's method of birth

Table 10.1 Inherited and acquired hypercoagulable states

ABNORMALITY	ARTERIAL VERSUS VENOUS	INCIDENCE IN NORMAL POPULATION	INCIDENCE IN PATIENTS WITH A FIRST VTE	INCIDENCE IN STROKE OR CAD PATIENTS	RISK OF VTE (APPROXIMATE)	RECURRENCE RATE	TREATMENT AFTER FIRST VTE
Heterozygous ATIII deficiency	Venous	0.2%	1%	Not increased	1.6% per year	60% lifetime	Life-long warfarin (INR 2.0–3.0).
Heterozygous protein C deficiency	Venous	0.3%	3%	Not increased	1% per year	60% lifetime	Individualize.
Heterozygous protein S deficiency	Venous ? Arterial	1% (when defined by low *free* protein S)	1%	Possibly increased	0.4% per year	60% lifetime risk in affected families; 30% in sporadic cases	Sporadic: warfarin for 6 months. Familial: individualize.
Heterozygous factor V Leiden (Arg^{506} → Gln) mutation	Venous ? MI	5% White 2% Hispanic 1% Black 0.5% Asian	12%: age 40–60 26%: age >60	MI possibly increased in women smokers	0.1–0.2% per year until age 69 0.6% per year over age 70	50% lifetime	Individualize.
Prothrombin G20210A	Venous ? Arterial	2%	6%	Possibly increased	Probably 0.1% per year (= risk in unaffected)	Probably 50% lifetime	Individualize.
Hyperhomocystinemia (fasting level >18.5 μmol/L)	Venous and arterial	5%	10%	18% of MI, stroke, or peripheral arterial patients under age 45	Not known	Not known	Warfarin for 6 months. Folic acid + vitamin B$_6$ + vitamin B$_{12}$ will reduce levels.
Antiphospholipid antibody	Venous and arterial	1%	10%	Increased ~10% lifetime risk of suffering a stroke	1% per year	23% per year	Life-long warfarin targeted to INR 3.0–3.5.
Previous venous thromboembolism	Venous	—	—	Not increased	—	30% at 8 years	Warfarin for 6 months. Vigorous prophylaxis in high-risk settings.

Table 10.1 Continued

ABNORMALITY	ARTERIAL VERSUS VENOUS	INCIDENCE IN NORMAL POPULATION	INCIDENCE IN PATIENTS WITH A FIRST VTE	INCIDENCE IN STROKE OR CAD PATIENTS	RISK OF VTE (APPROXIMATE)	RECURRENCE RATE	TREATMENT AFTER FIRST VTE
Oral contraceptives (OCs)	Venous	—	50% of women age 15–49	Not increased	0.4% per year	High if OCs not discontinued	Stop OCs. Warfarin for 6 months.
Prior surgery	Venous	—	18%	Not increased	50%: orthopedic[a] 30%: urologic[a] 30%: abdominal[a]	—	Warfarin for 6 months.
Trauma	Venous	—	—	Not increased	>50%: pelvic, hip, head, or spinal cord	—	Inferior vena cava filter or warfarin for 6 months.
Cancer	Venous	2% (over age 60)	10%	Not increased	Not known	High	Individualize.
Immobilization	Venous	1%	15%	Not increased	Increased	—	Warfarin for 6 months.
Pregnancy	Venous	—	—	Not increased	0.6% per year (10-fold increase over age-matched women)	—	Heparin until postpartum. Then warfarin for 6 months.
Hormone replacement therapy (HRT)	Venous	—	—	Not increased	0.4% per year	Not known	? Warfarin for 6 months. Stop HRT.
Nephrotic syndrome	Venous—adults Arterial—children	—	—	Pediatric stroke and mesenteric and limb ischemia/infarction	20% lifetime risk	High	Individualize.
Age	Venous and arterial	—	—	Increased	0.01% age 40 0.10% age 55 1.00% age 75	—	Warfarin for 6 months.

[a] Without prophylaxis.

Abbreviations: CAD = coronary artery disease; INR = international normalized ratio; MI = myocardial infarction; VTE = venous thromboembolism.

control away from an oral contraceptive when it is associated with venous thromboembolism.

As more and more genetic thrombophilias associated with VTE are recognized, more and more ambiguities about their optimal treatment emerge. The most important question we must ask is this: Should the patient be on life-long warfarin anticoagulation? To answer the question, we must consider the therapeutic index of warfarin for each individual patient who is being considered for this type of treatment. Under the best of conditions, targeting an INR of 2.0–3.0 (1), there is about a 4% per year risk of nonfatal major hemorrhage. And what are the benefits of extending warfarin beyond 6 months? In patients suffering a first symptomatic DVT *without* an identified hypercoagulable state and with no obvious trigger, there is a recurrence risk of 17% at 2 years, 25% at 5 years, and 30% at 8 years (2); there is evidence that the recurrence rate is decreased by 95% in patients receiving long-term warfarin anticoagulation (1). The recurrence risk is also decreased when there is a triggering event that is eliminated, but we do not yet know when such an intervention (e.g., stopping oral contraceptives) absolutely precludes the need for long-term anticoagulation. Similarly, although the impact of an inherited thrombophilia on recurrence rate is generally unfavorable, we do not yet know which thrombophilias absolutely require life-long anticoagulation.

Table 10.1 presents a summary of current information about the epidemiology of acquired and inherited hypercoagulable states, and some recommendations about treatment. If the treatment recommendations are ambiguous or vague, it is intentional. Better recommendations will soon be available, based on the results of the ongoing U.S. PREVENT (Prevention of Venous Thromboembolism) and Canadian ELATE (Extended Low Intensity Anticoagulation in Idiopathic Thromboembolism) clinical trials.

Who Should Be Evaluated?

Not everyone who presents with VTE should receive a hypercoagulable workup. Current recommendations are provided by Dr. Ken Bauer (6), who suggests that all patients who are "strongly" thrombophilic be tested. He defines strongly thrombophilic as those whose thrombosis occurred before age 50, those who have had recurrent thromboses, *or* those with a family history of thrombosis ("weakly" thrombophilic patients are those without any of these clinical characteristics). In addition, persons with thromboses in unusual sites should be evaluated.

Mesenteric thrombosis occurs more commonly in patients with antithrombin III deficiency, protein S deficiency, or protein C deficiency, and in association with prothrombin G20210A. Prothrombin G20210A also is associated with cerebral vein thrombosis. Patients with hepatic-vein thrombosis, *Budd-Chiari syndrome*, should be evaluated for the underlying myeloproliferative disorder polycythemia vera or paroxysmal nocturnal hemoglobinuria. Patients with renal vein thrombosis should be evaluated for the nephrotic syndrome. The upper extremities are *not* considered an unusual site.

Table 10.2   Laboratory evaluation for strongly thrombophilic patients

- Screen for resistance to activated protein C (APC) by clotting assay or genetic test for factor V-Arg^{506} → Gln (factor V Leiden).
  Confirm positive APC resistance assay with genetic test.
- Genetic test for prothrombin G20210A mutation.
- Functional assay of antithrombin III (heparin-cofactor assay).[a]
- Functional assay of protein C.[a]
- Functional assay of protein S along with immunological assays of total and free protein S.[a]
- Clotting assay for lupus anticoagulant and ELISA for antiphospholipid antibodies
- Measurement of fasting total plasma homocysteine levels

[a] Omit in "weakly" thrombophilic patients as deficiencies of antithrombin III, protein C, or protein S are very infrequently identified.

Reproduced by permission from Bauer KA. Update on thrombophilia. Hematology 1999: The Educational Program of the American Society of Hematology: 233–234.

Laboratory Evaluation

Table 10.2 lists the type of laboratory workup that can be applied to patients who are "strongly" thrombophilic. An understanding of the limitations of testing is required to prevent false-positive results. Most importantly, it is essential that the presence of VTE is documented objectively. It is also essential that testing only be performed either immediately (before any anticoagulation is started) or a few weeks after the full course of treatment has been completed. This is because heparin will affect the antithrombin III levels, whereas warfarin will affect the protein C and protein S levels.

Protein S levels are particularly tricky to measure because they are affected by many conditions. Protein S circulates in a free (about 40%) and bound (about 60%) state. Binding is to the acute phase C4-binding protein, and bound protein S is inactive. Free protein S therefore drops in inflammatory states. Total protein S increases with age, waxes and wanes with the menstrual cycle, decreases in patients who are pregnant or taking oral contraceptives, and can be decreased during an acute VTE episode. For antithrombin III and protein C, a single activity value of greater than 50% *off anticoagulant therapy* is a reliable diagnostic result to rule out the deficient state. A value less than 50% on at least two separate measurements confirms the diagnosis of antithrombin III deficiency or protein C deficiency. For protein S, one should measure activity and quantify free and bound protein on at least two occasions before making any conclusions about a deficiency state.

Homocysteine levels vary with diet and should be measured in the fasting state. Homocysteine levels after methionine loading may identify more hyper-homocystinemic persons, but the clinical relevance of provoked positive test results is unknown and such testing is not recommended. Tests for factor V Leiden and prothrombin G20210A are simple PCR-based assays of the mutant germline DNA sequence that can be performed at any time on a person's DNA from any source.

About 20% of activated protein C (APC) resistant states are *not* associated with the factor V Leiden mutation, and therefore rely on the functional assay. The functional assay for APC resistance is reasonably well standardized, but still requires an experienced operator to establish the standard curves and measure the deficiency. In the best assay currently available, the patient's plasma is diluted 1:5 with factor V–deficient plasma. An aPTT is generated on this specimen. The aPTT is then measured on this same specimen to which is added activated protein C. The activated protein C will break down the normal factors V and VIII in the specimen and thereby prolong the aPTT. When a patient is APC deficient, the breakdown is prevented (for example, by the mutant $Arg^{506} \rightarrow Gln$ cleavage site) and the prolongation of the aPTT is decreased. APC resistance is defined by a patient's aPTT prolonging less than 20% of the control.

Inherited Syndromes

Antithrombin III (ATIII) Deficiency

ATIII (also designated simply as *antithrombin*) is a natural anticoagulant that inactivates factor X and thrombin (see Chapter 1). ATIII deficiency results from over 80 different mutations in the ATIII gene transmitted in an autosomal dominant fashion. These mutations usually decrease the amount of functional protein (type I deficiency), although some cause a normal quantity of dysfunctional protein (type II deficiency). The homozygous state is lethal. The heterozygous state is diagnosed by measuring a level of ATIII less than 50% on two separate occasions. Heparin, disseminated intravascular coagulation (DIC), oral contraceptives, cirrhosis, and the nephrotic syndrome decrease ATIII levels. ATIII levels are sometimes increased by warfarin. The heterozygous state has been observed in up to 0.2% of normal people unaffected by VTE, 1% of those with a first VTE, and 4% of affected persons with a first-degree relative with VTE.

The life-long risk of recurrence is quite high (60% to 80%), and most experts would seriously consider life-long anticoagulation following a first VTE in someone who has heterozygous ATIII deficiency. An ATIII concentrate is available, but there are currently no proven indications for its use. In general, its use should be considered in ATIII-deficient patients with "heparin resistance" or to facilitate VTE prophylaxis in patients at high risk for both thrombosis and hemorrhage, such as with neurosurgical trauma and obstetrical surgery.

Dosing of ATIII Concentrates
1. Each milliliter of ATIII concentrate has 1 U of activity.
2. The volume of distribution is the intravascular compartment.
3. The target level is 100%.
4. The half-life is 48 hours.

5. For a 50-kg person whose ATIII level is 40%: infuse 60 U/kg = 3000 U distributed in an intravascular compartment volume of about 4.5 liters (0.67 U/mL final concentration) for an increase in ATIII level to about 107% (0.4 U/mL beginning concentration [40%] + 0.67 U/mL infused [67%] concentration = 1.07 U/mL [107%] final concentration).

6. Maintenance therapy can begin with 60% of the starting dose given every 24 hours.

7. Monitor levels daily and adjust maintenance dose or schedule to maintain an 80% (0.8 U/mL) level.

8. Stop ATIII when heparin is discontinued or when the crisis resolves.

Protein C Deficiency

Protein C (PC) is a vitamin K–dependent natural anticoagulant protein that inactivates factors V and VIII. PC deficiency results from over 160 different mutations. Heterozygous PC deficiency is inherited in an autosomal dominant pattern. Like ATIII, it is classified as type I (quantitative deficiency) or type II (qualitative dysfunction). The heterozygous state results in levels of activity less than 50%. Liver disease, DIC, sepsis, and chemotherapy (particularly asparaginase) also decrease PC activity. PC activity is not decreased by the nephrotic syndrome.

The most important clinical factor that causes reduced PC levels is warfarin therapy. When warfarin therapy begins in patients who are not receiving heparin, there is a transient imbalance in the procoagulant/anticoagulant axis (see Chapter 1) with a relative deficiency in PC because it has a very short half-life (about 6 hours, similar to factor VII) compared with factors II, IX, and X (72, 24, and 36 hours, respectively). In a patient with PC deficiency, this imbalance is amplified and can lead to acute thrombosis in the veins and venules of the skin of the arms, breasts, trunk, and penis. This *warfarin-induced skin necrosis* is rare, but when it develops in persons who are deficient in PC it improves only when PC is repleted by fresh frozen plasma infusion. Heterozygous PC deficiency will lead to VTE in over 60% of affected individuals, but the VTEs rarely develop before the age of 20, and then the risk increases during each progressive decade of life. In contrast, homozygous PC deficiency is a severe disease of the fetus and neonate called "purpura fulminans." This is treatable with fresh frozen plasma or protein C concentrates (not yet commercially available).

Protein S Deficiency

Protein S (PS) deficiency is transmitted as an autosomal dominant condition. It results from over 60 mutations in the gene for PS. PS measurements are confounded by binding to C4-binding protein, which affects the active free PS concentration (see above). It is therefore difficult to establish precisely the incidence of heterozygous PS deficiency, although (as listed in Table 10.1) it is quite common when defined by a free PS level less than 50%. Most experts think that free PS activity measurements are often false positive, and that any PS deficiency suspected because of a low free PS measurement must be confirmed by measuring total and free PS protein on at least two occasions.

Because of the variability of measurements of PS, it is difficult to establish a tight correlation of PS level with risk of first VTE, recurrent VTE, or arterial thrombosis. A family history is perhaps the most reliable factor, indicating a true pathogenetic link between an individual with PS deficiency and VTE. In a patient with a first VTE, PS deficiency, and no family history of VTE, routine treatment is indicated. Patients with a family history may be at increased risk of recurrence, and one should examine the risks and benefits of more long-term anticoagulation therapy for such individuals.

Factor V Leiden

Factor V Leiden results from a point mutation in codon 506. This point mutation causes an arginine residue to be replaced with a glutamine, resulting in factor V resistance to breakdown by activated protein C. The heterozygous state is quite common in certain regions (perhaps 15% of all people in Southern Spain and 4% of people in the Netherlands), but is uncommon in Hispanics, Africans, African-Americans, Asians, Indians, and Middle Eastern people. In whites, the presence of a single allele of factor V Leiden increases the risk of a first VTE sevenfold, whereas homozygosity increases the risk 80-fold. Risk is greatest for DVT, cerebral vein thrombosis, and superficial venous thrombosis, and less so for PE; the risk is probably absent for retinal vein thrombosis and arterial thrombosis. In fact, heterozygous factor V Leiden is by far the most commonly identified abnormality when patients are tested after suffering a first DVT. It is found in almost 20% of first DVT patients without a family history, and perhaps 40% of those with a family history of DVT.

Factor V Leiden is common enough that there is ample clinical experience to demonstrate that it synergizes with other risk factors (see below). Only in these cases should life-long warfarin anticoagulation be considered. Approximately 20% of all APC resistance is not associated with factor V Leiden. If you observe a positive functional assay for APC resistance and a negative molecular assay for factor V Leiden, the recurrence risk is probably relatively low (less than factor V Leiden) and use of long-term anticoagulation therapy should be avoided. APC resistance without factor V Leiden may, however, be a risk factor for arterial vaso-occlusive diseases.

Prothrombin 20210 Mutation

The prothrombin 20210 point mutation in the 3′ noncoding region of the prothrombin gene causes a glycine residue to be converted to an alanine. By some yet unknown mechanism, the mutation causes levels of prothrombin (factor II) to increase by 15% or greater. The way that factor II levels of 115%

increase risk for VTE and cerebral vein thrombosis (and perhaps arterial thrombosis) is not yet known, but it raises many interesting questions about the fine-tuning of the hemostatic/thrombotic balance and serves as a reminder that factor replacement therapy (see Chapter 17) must avoid overshooting normal physiological levels.

The prothrombin 20210 mutation causes a twofold to threefold increased risk of a first VTE. The risk of recurrence is increased to almost 50%, but there are no established data that long-term warfarin anticoagulation should be used when the prothrombin 20210 mutation is the only risk factor identified in patients with a first VTE.

Mixed Syndrome

Hyperhomocystinemia

Genetic factors, dietary factors, and other factors such as (particularly) smoking regulate blood levels of homocysteine (7). Mild (and worse) hyperhomocystinemia appears to directly injure vascular endothelium, leading to an increased risk of both VTE and arterial thrombosis. The genetic disorder homocystinuria, caused by the deficiency of the enzyme cystathionine β-synthase, leads to extremely high hyperhomocystinemia and is associated with severe premature atherosclerosis and VTE.

Mild hyperhomocystinemia (defined as a fasting plasma level of $> 18.5\,\mu M$) can be found in 5% to 10% of healthy adults. Mild hyperhomocystinemia is observed in about 10% to 15% of all patients with a first VTE (8) and is associated with a twofold increased risk of recurrence. It is also observed in up to 40% of patients with coronary and/or cerebral atherosclerosis, and should be considered when evaluating young patients with symptomatic coronary heart disease and stroke. Unlike homocystinemia, no specific genetic abnormality has yet to be related to mild homocystinemia, and it appears that most cases are related to diet, vitamin intake, and smoking rather than heredity. A common mutation of the methylenetetrahydrofolate reductase gene affecting up to 10% of the general population has been described, which leads to mild hyperhomocystinemia without associated VTE. The basis for this apparent paradox is at this time unknown.

High levels of homocysteine can be decreased by vitamin supplementation, particularly with folic acid. Levels can often be further decreased by vitamins B_6 and B_{12} supplementation. The effect on the natural history of VTE and on atherosclerotic arterial diseases of reducing homocysteine levels is not yet established. Nevertheless, it is reasonable to prescribe these vitamins to patients with mild hyperhomocystinemia associated with such diseases, as they are safe and inexpensive. If vitamins are used, it is important to measure homocysteine levels and target the reduction to less than $15\,\mu M$ total plasma homocysteine. Firm data on outcome, optimal dosing, and optimal target homocysteine levels should become available within the next 5 to 10 years.

Acquired Syndromes

Antiphospholipid (APL) Syndrome

The antiphospholipid (APL) syndrome is discussed in Chapter 9. In a patient with a VTE or arterial thrombosis (most commonly stroke) associated with an APL, long-term anticoagulation should target an INR of 3.0–3.5. If the APL is secondary due to a condition that is in remission, it should be remeasured; if it has disappeared, one can consider stopping warfarin. Similarly, in a patient with a primary APL syndrome who has been treated for over 1 year, it is reasonable to recheck the APL titer and, if it is gone, consider stopping warfarin.

Previous Thrombosis

A DVT damages the vessel wall and creates an increased risk of recurrent DVT. Of interest, not all recurrences are ipsilateral (2). This suggests that there may be occult injury of the contralateral femoral venous system transmitted by the effects of abnormal flow in the inferior vena caval circuit. The clinical manifestations of the "postphlebitic syndrome" are difficult to distinguish from recurrent ipsilateral DVT. Similarly, noninvasive studies are generally not useful unless one directly compares the flow and ultrasound characteristics to those while the patient was in a clinical remission.

Because of these diagnostic difficulties and the well-established risk of ipsilateral recurrence in the absence of any other hypercoagulable factor, some practitioners treat these patients with routine heparin therapy followed by indefinite warfarin anticoagulation. I suggest that this is a situation in which one should use contrast venography, and life-long warfarin anticoagulation should be considered only for those patients whose venograms unequivocally demonstrate fresh thrombi. Patients with a previous VTE should receive vigorous prophylaxis during risk periods, including outpatient prophylaxis.

Oral Contraceptives

Oral contraceptives are the most common cause of VTE among the women who use them. Oral contraceptives also synergize with other risk factors. Even with doses of ethinyl estradiol of less than 50 µg, the procoagulant/anticoagulant balance is tipped in favor of thrombosis, and there is a fourfold increased risk of VTE. There appears to be an unexpected jump in risk of VTE associated with newer progestational agents added to oral contraceptives, in part because these agents mysteriously cause acquired APC resistance.

When a patient who has been taking oral contraceptives develops a VTE, the medication should be stopped, alternative birth control implemented, and routine anticoagulation prescribed. If the woman stays off oral contraceptives, the risk of recurrence is significantly decreased below that of normal persons after a first VTE without any obvious trigger.

Surgery

The risk for VTE in patients undergoing surgery without prophylaxis is approximately 50% for a broken femur or tibia, 40% for a total hip or knee replacement or a total prostatectomy, 30% for major abdominal surgery, 25% for neurosurgery, 20% for gynecological surgery, and 10% for transurethral procedures. The risk is significantly decreased with prophylactic anticoagulation; however, even in these patients about 5% to 10% will develop a calf vein or proximal DVT, and the postoperative state is associated with 18% of first VTEs even when good prophylaxis is given.

Trauma

Multiple trauma is associated with a 50% risk of having VTE. Prophylaxis reduces this by about 75%. Prophylaxis is individualized: low-molecular-weight heparin is effective *and safe* even in patients with brain or spinal cord trauma, but nonpharmacological prophylaxis with intermittent external pneumatic leg compression is equally effective and eliminates any risk of hemorrhage. Treatment of an acute VTE in this setting is rarely routine, and often an inferior vena cava filter is the only predictably safe and effective treatment program. When anticoagulation therapy can be administered, routine heparin followed by 6 months of warfarin is the standard program.

Cancer

The association of cancer and VTE is well documented. Patients with cancer are at increased risk of VTE, even when they are active outpatients. The risk is not easily quantified, but estimates are that cancer increases the risk fivefold. *Trousseau's syndrome* is migratory superficial thrombophlebitis that develops in some patients with cancer, particularly adenocarcinomas of the lung, colon, and pancreas. VTE is, however, a far more common (if not less dramatic) sign of occult malignancy.

Among all patients with a first VTE, a new malignancy is diagnosed in about 12%. The diagnosis is usually made at presentation (9), but when a cancer is not initially diagnosed but then emerges, it emerges within 6 months of the presenting VTE episode (10). This has led some practitioners to emphasize that the most important hypercoagulable state to evaluate for patients with VTE is an occult malignancy. Fortunately, such an evaluation requires no more than the routine workup undertaken for all patients who suffer an acute illness: history, examination, screening blood work, and a good PA and lateral chest x-ray (9,10).

Immobilization

Immobilization is a risk factor for VTE, although it is probably less than popularly thought. In the Leiden Thrombophilia Study, 15.6% of all first VTE patients had a history of immobilization at some time *within the past 1 year.*

Immobilization need not be in a hospital bed, and there are anecdotes of VTE associated with air travel and even traffic jams. Be aware that homebound patients who are immobilized may be at risk just as much as a patient in the coronary care unit, so adequate prophylaxis should be considered for in-home settings.

Pregnancy

The risk of VTE during pregnancy is about 0.5 per 1000 women. This is over 10-fold the risk of nonpregnant age-matched controls. Most studies show that the risk during the puerperium is much greater than before delivery. It is therefore reasonable to give heparin prophylaxis to all women who are bed-bound in anticipation of delivery, or to those who suffer postpartum complications causing immobilization. In women with previous pregnancy-related VTE, prophylactic low-molecular-weight heparin is often given during the entire pregnancy, followed by warfarin anticoagulation for 4 to 6 weeks after the birth. Recent data challenge this approach (see Chapter 19).

Estrogen Replacement Therapy

Postmenopausal hormone therapy increases the risk of VTE twofold to fourfold. The risk is not substantially less than that of oral contraceptive use, demonstrating that the risk-threshold concentration of estrogens is lower than expected. Hormone replacement therapy (HRT) adds to the risk of VTE in women who have other acquired risk factors such as hip fracture, surgery, or cancer. There is evidence that aspirin given to women who have coronary artery disease actually decreases the risk of HRT-associated VTE (11).

Age

Age is an important risk factor. In the absence of any other risk factors, VTE occurs infrequently in persons under the age of 40 (<1 per 10,000) and frequently in persons over the age of 75 (>1 per 100), with a fairly steady geometric increase in risk associated with age over 40. The effect of age must be considered when examining the association between VTE and other risk factors.

Miscellaneous

The *nephrotic syndrome*, probably because it results in the loss of ATIII in the urine, is associated with thrombosis, particularly of the renal vein (up to 30%) and the deep leg veins (up to 25%). *The myeloproliferative disorders*—polycythemia vera, essential thrombocytosis, and paroxysmal nocturnal hemoglobinuria—are associated with thrombosis. The natural history of untreated polycythemia vera frequently involves thrombosis, with 40% of all deaths related to either VTE or acute arterial occlusion syndromes. Most arterial thromboses in polycythemia vera are related to hyperviscosity. When phlebotomy is used to normalize the hematocrit, mortality from myocardial infarction and stroke are greatly reduced, although the risk of suffering from VTE remains about 20%. The current standard treatment for polycythemia vera is hydroxyurea, and this form of chemical cytoreduction greatly reduces the risk of VTE, although one must be vigilant for the onset of VTE in all patients with polycythemia vera, no matter how monotonous the blood profile becomes.

Essential thrombocytosis (ET) is associated with both venous and arterial thrombosis, although arterial thromboses are more common. Hydroxyurea targeting a platelet count below 600,000/µL appears to minimize the risk of arterial vaso-occlusion in patients with a history of and/or significant risks for arterial thrombosis (see Chapter 11).

Paroxysmal nocturnal hemoglobinuria (PNH) is a clonal myeloid disorder resulting in an acquired defect in the synthesis of a *phosphatidylinositol glycan* that anchors many cell surface proteins, including several complement inhibitory proteins. Patients with PNH have red cells that are unusually susceptible to complement-induced damage, and PNH platelets become activated by the unbalanced activation of the complement cascade on their surface. However, the pathophysiology of thrombosis in PNH isn't as simple as hyperactive platelets, as PNH patients are probably more susceptible to venous than arterial thromboses.

Myeloproliferative disorders can be associated with two rare but distinctive clinical syndromes: erythromelalgia and the Budd-Chiari syndrome. Erythromelalgia is an inflammatory disease (pain, redness, swelling) of the toes and/or fingers resulting from ischemia from very high platelet counts or, less commonly, very high hematocrits. It usually responds to antiplatelet therapy and cytoreduction. Budd-Chiari syndrome is due to acute hepatic vein thrombosis. It can be a devastating condition, leading to liver swelling, pain, and dysfunction. It is most commonly associated with polycythemia vera or PNH, but can be a complication of virtually every condition listed in Table 10.1. It is diagnosed by contrast venography or MRI, although duplex ultrasonography can sometimes reveal the hepatic vein thrombus. Budd-Chiari syndrome is best treated by thrombolytic therapy followed by heparin and warfarin.

As described above, the common prothrombin G20210A mutation appears to cause VTE because blood levels of prothrombin are elevated to 115% or greater. Similarly, elevated levels of *factor VIII*, *factor XI*, and *fibrinogen* appear to be real risk factors for venous thrombosis. Factor VIII levels are constitutionally elevated above 150% in about 10% of the population, and such an elevation is associated with a twofold to threefold increase in risk for VTE. Although factor VIII levels rise when its carrier protein von Willebrand factor is nonspecifically elevated due to inflammation, elevated von Willebrand factor does not appear to cause a hypercoagulable state. Factor XI levels above the 90th percentile (about 121%) are found in about 10% of the white population, and such levels increase the risk of VTE twofold. Fibrinogen levels are somewhat more variable over a larger range than are prothrombin, factor VIII, or factor XI levels. Nonetheless, relative elevations of plasma fibrinogen (within the normal range) appear to be a risk factor for both venous and arterial thrombosis. The mechanism by which elevated procoagulant proteins increase the risk for thrombosis is not known, and there are no treatments for these conditions.

In contrast, it is easy to understand how vascular *catheters* make one hypercoagulable: both the blood vessel and blood flow are adversely affected. Vascular catheters are the most common reason for thrombosis in a pediatric population. In adults, daily low-dose warfarin (1 mg) can prevent catheter-related thrombosis.

Synergistic Risk

Factor V Leiden synergizes with other risk factors, including oral contraceptives, prothrombin G20210A mutation, hyperhomocystinemia, and deficiencies of protein C and S. For example, if factor V Leiden and oral contraceptives are individually associated with a fourfold increased risk of VTE, together they increase the risk 30-fold. Oral contraceptives and mutant prothrombin probably also synergize with other risk factors and each other, although there is evidence that prothrombin G20210A does not cause a synergistic risk of VTE in persons deficient in protein C. The observation that individuals with two genetic risk factors experience a greater than additive increase in recurrent VTE is the basis for the recommendation that such patients be considered for long-term warfarin anticoagulation after a first VTE (see below).

Management

Hypercoagulable patients with VTE should be managed according to Table 10.3. Screening asymptomatic family members is currently not recommended. When an asymptomatic person is discovered to carry a hypercoagulable trait, that person should be counseled about the symptoms of VTE, how to use VTE prophylaxis during risk periods, and about how contraceptives affect risk. Screening for the common genetic factors factor V Leiden and prothrombin G20210A is not currently recommended before starting women on oral contraceptives. It is reasonable, however, to inquire about a family history of VTE before prescribing oral contraceptives, and to test those with a first-degree relative with a *documented* DVT or PE. All patients with antiphospholipid antibodies (APAs) require indefinite warfarin targeted to an INR of 3.0–3.5. Otherwise, warfarin is given targeting an INR of 2.0–3.0, and it is reasonable to use a target INR of 2.0 for patients who expect to receive life-long anticoagulation.

All hypercoagulable patients (except APL patients) with arterial thrombosis should receive antiplatelet therapy (see Chapter 9). Combined antiplatelet and warfarin therapy should only be used for patients with both arterial and venous thrombosis who fail to respond to a single agent. When both antiplatelet and

Table 10.3   Management of hypercoagulable patients with VTE

RISK CLASSIFICATION	MANAGEMENT
High Risk	
2 or more spontaneous events	Indefinite management
• 1 spontaneous life-threatening event (near-fatal pulmonary embolus, cerebral, mesenteric, or portal vein thrombosis)	
• 1 spontaneous event in association with antiphospholipid antibody syndrome, antithrombin III deficiency, or more than one genetic defect	
Moderate Risk	
• 1 event with a known provocative stimulus	Vigorous prophylaxis in high-risk settings
• Asymptomatic	

Reproduced by permission from Bauer KA. Update on thrombophilia. Hematology 1999: The Educational Program of the American Society of Hematology:233–234.

warfarin therapy are used together, the patient must be monitored very carefully for bleeding.

Annotated Bibliography

1. Kearon C, Gent M, Hirsh J, et al. A comparison of three months of anticoagulation with extended anticoagulation for a first episode of idiopathic venous thromboembolism. N Engl J Med 1999;340:901–907.

   In this study, 162 patients with idiopathic VTE who had completed 3 months of warfarin were randomized to treatment with warfarin (targeted to an INR of 2.0–3.0) or placebo. The mean duration of follow-up was 10 months. Of 83 patients treated with placebo, 17 had VTE recurrence, whereas there was only 1 recurrence out of 79 warfarin-treated patients. Nonfatal major bleeding occurred in 3 out of 79 warfarin-treated patients. How should patients be treated, and for how long after the 3-month period? This study recommends at least 3 months at an INR of 2.0–3.0, and perhaps (much) longer at a lower INR, whatever the risk factor profile. This question may be better answered by the PREVENT or ELATE trials, and the reader should watch for their published reports.

2. Prandoni P, Lensing AWA, Cogo A, et al. The long-term clinical course of acute deep venous thrombosis. Ann Intern Med 1996;125:1–7.

   In this study, 355 consecutive patients with the diagnosis of symptomatic DVT were followed after routine treatment (usually heparin followed by 3 months of warfarin targeted to an INR of 2.0–3.0); 78 patients had a recurrence: 35 ipsilateral DVT, 28 contralateral DVT, and 15 PE (9 of which were fatal). The cumulative incidence of recurrence was 17.5% at 2 years, 24.6% at 5 years, and 30.3% at 8 years. The cumulative incidence of the postphlebitic (or *post-thrombotic*) syndrome was 22.8% at 2 years, 28% at 5 years, and 29.1% at 8 years. Patients with postphlebitic syndrome were at greatest risk for ipsilateral recurrence.

3. Sanson BJ, Simioni P, Tormene D, et al. The incidence of venous thromboembolism in asymptomatic carriers of a deficiency of antithrombin, protein C, or protein S: a prospective cohort study. Blood 1999;94:3702–3706.

A cohort of *asymptomatic* young individuals with familial deficiencies of antithrombin III, protein C, and protein S was followed for the development of DVT. Each person was given routine prophylaxis during periods on increased risk for VTE, but otherwise no interventions were prescribed. The annual incidence of VTE was 1.6% for antithrombin-deficient, 1.0% for protein C-deficient, and 0.4% for protein S–deficient individuals. It was concluded that preemptive anticoagulation therapy is inappropriate in such high-risk patients.

4. Ridker PM, Glynn RJ, Miletich JP, et al. Age-specific incidence rates of venous thromboembolism among heterozygous carriers of factor V Lieden mutation. Ann Intern Med 1997;126:528–531.

The incidence rates of VTE associated with factor V Leiden among members of the Physicians Health Study jumped up dramatically after age 70. This suggests that age synergizes with factor V Leiden as risk factors for VTE and reminds us that hypercoagulability is not limited to young persons.

5. Simioni P, Prandoni P, Lensing AWA, et al. The risk of recurrent venous thromboembolism in patients with an Arg^{506} → Gln mutation in the gene for factor V (factor V Leiden). N Engl J Med 1997;336:399–403.

Factor V Leiden was associated with a cumulative incidence of recurrence of 40% compared to a 18% cumulative incidence for those with a first episode VTE without factor V Leiden.

6. Bauer KA. Update on Thrombophilia in Hematology 1999: The Educational Program of the American Society of Hematology (ASH). Washington, DC: American Society of Hematology, 1999:231–235.

A concise practical review written by a long-standing leader in the field.

7. D'Angelo A, Selhub J. Homocysteine and thrombotic disease. Blood 1997;90:1–11.

A thorough review of the biochemistry and pathophysiology of homocysteine.

8. Fermo I, D'Angelo SV, Paroni R, et al. Prevalence of moderate hyperhomocysteinemia in patients with early-onset venous and arterial occlusive disease. Ann Intern Med 1995;123:747–753.

Fasting and provoked hyperhomocystinemia were examined in 107 patients with VTE and 50 patients with arterial disease. All patients were younger than 45 years old. Fasting hyperhomocystinemia was defined as greater than 15 μM (females) or greater than 19.5 μM (males). It was detected in 13% of patients with VTE and 19% of patients with arterial vaso-occlusive diseases. Hyperhomocystinemia affected 26 of the 30 patient families studied.

9. Cornuz J, Pearson SD, Creager MA, et al. Importance of findings on the initial evaluation for cancer in patients with symptomatic idiopathic deep venous thrombosis. Ann Intern Med 1996;125:785–793.

Cancer was diagnosed in 12% of 136 hospitalized patients with DVT. All of the patients discovered to have cancer had the diagnosis made by the routine evaluation at the time of admission for DVT: history, physical examination, basic laboratory testing, and chest x-ray. When a routine workup failed to reveal cancer, all DVT patients had a risk of developing cancer equal to the healthy controls.

10. Sorensen HT, Mellemkjaer L, Steffensen FH, et al. The risk of a diagnosis of cancer after primary deep venous thrombosis or pulmonary embolism. N Engl J Med 1998;338:1169–1222.

Two very large cohorts of Danish patients with DVT (15,348) or PE (11,305) were followed for developing cancer simultaneously or after the diagnosis of VTE. Cancer was diagnosed in 11.3% and 6.4% of patients with DVT and PE, respectively. The relative risk of diagnosing cancer was modestly increased: a standardized incidence ratio of 1.3 for both DVT and PE. The diagnosis was usually made within 6 months of VTE using a routine workup. The standardized incidence ratio fell to just slightly more than 1.0 one year after the diagnosis of VTE. The most common associated cancers were pancreatic, ovarian, hepatocellular, and brain. In many cases, establishing the association between VTE and cancer had no effect on the natural history of the cancer: 40% of all cancers were metastatic at the time of diagnosis.

11. Grady D, Wenger NK, Herrington D, et al. Postmenopausal hormone therapy increases risk for venous thromboembolic disease. The Heart and Estrogen/progestin Replacement Study. Ann Intern Med 2000;132:689–696.

The Heart and Estrogen/progestin Replacement Study (HERS) randomized 2763 postmenopausal women under 80 years old to receive daily conjugated equine estrogen (0.625 mg) plus medroxyprogesterone acetate (2.5 mg), or placebo. There were 34 women in the treatment arm and 13 women in the placebo arm who had VTE. The risk of VTE was increased to 3.9 women out of 1000 per year. Risk was increased by leg fracture, cancer, inpatient surgery, or nonsurgical hospitalization. Risk was decreased by aspirin or statin therapy.

11

Thrombocytosis

An elevated platelet count is always important. Thrombocytosis either is a sign of an underlying disease (*secondary thrombocytosis*) or is itself a disease process associated with a distinctive natural history that includes an increased risk of thrombosis (*essential thrombocytosis* or *thrombocythemia*).

Differential Diagnosis

The criteria for diagnosing the myeloproliferative disorder essential thrombocytosis (ET) are listed in Table 11.1. They provide a good perspective from which to approach the diagnostic evaluation for any patient with thrombocytosis. They also demonstrate that ET is a diagnosis of exclusion, with the immediate task faced by the physician being to ensure that the elevated platelet count is not a sign of an underlying disease, particularly another myeloproliferative disorder or an occult malignancy. To rule out an occult malignancy, one simply employs a routine workup, including history, physical examination, chest x-ray, and laboratory studies (including prostate-specific antigen in men). When an occult malignancy is excluded, one then considers iron deficiency, hemolysis, or bleeding, any of which can result in a reactive thrombocytosis. An occult chronic inflammatory disease may be identified by measuring a C reactive protein, with the precise etiological entity pinpointed by focusing the laboratory evaluation on any subtle symptoms or signs that suggest a chronic rheumatologic, gastrointestinal, or infectious process.

Pathophysiology

The regulation of platelet production involves several growth factors and the interaction between growth factor–stimulated stem cells and stroma in the bone marrow environment. The growth factor that appears to be most important is thrombopoietin, but other growth factors and cytokines enhance platelet production (including interleukin-11, which is approved for use in the United States for chemotherapy-induced thrombocytopenia). It is therefore surprising that the

Table 11.1   Essential thrombocytosis diagnostic criteria

1. Platelet count > 600,000/μL.
2. Hematocrit < 40% of normal red cell mass (<36 mL/kg men; <32 mL/kg women). This rules out polycythemia vera.
3. Normal mean corpuscular volume or normal serum ferritin or marrow iron present. This rules out iron deficiency.
4. No bcr/abl fusion gene. This rules out chronic myelogenous leukemia.
5. Marrow biopsy fibrosis absent or <1/3 area without splenomegaly and leukoerythroblastic blood smear. This rules out myelofibrosis.
6. No clinical or cytogenetic evidence of a myelodysplastic disorder.
7. No cause for reactive thrombocytosis identified.

Source: Tefferi A. Risk-based management in essential thrombocythemia. In: Hematology 1999: American Society of Hematology education book. Washington, DC: American Society of Hematology, 1999:172–177.

cause of thrombocytosis (both ET and secondary thrombocytosis) is almost never related to alterations in blood thrombopoietin (TPO) levels or to abnormalities in the thrombopoietin receptor (designated c-mpl) found on megakaryocytes and platelets. Analyses of TPO and its receptor are therefore not useful for the diagnosis of thrombocytosis. It is perhaps equally surprising that at least one-quarter of patients with ET do not have a monoclonal proliferation of megakaryocytes. When considering such facts, it is hardly a revelation to characterize the cause of thrombocytosis as "unknown."

A solution to one of the mysteries of thrombocytosis is tantalizingly close: bleeding, hemolysis, and iron deficiency all stimulate the expression in hematopoietic stem cells of the DNA binding protein GATA-1. There is good evidence that GATA-1 regulates the transcription of both erythroid and megakaryocytic genes involved in proliferation and blood cell development, and this mechanism provides a reasonable model for the cause of elevated platelet counts in these clinical conditions.

Clinical Features

ET is uncommon, with about new 6000 diagnoses annually in the United States. ET appears to be twice as prevalent in women. It is rarely lethal: less than 5% of all cases terminate in leukemic transformation. Its natural history is not, however, benign—there can be severe morbidity related to thrombosis in almost one-half of cases if they go untreated. The incidence of secondary thrombocytosis is not known.

The risk of thrombosis in persons with secondary thrombocytosis is low and mainly unpredictable. The exception to this is venous thromboembolism (VTE) in patients who undergo splenectomy for immune hemolysis. In these patients, the efflux of excessive numbers of platelets and young red cells into the circulation leads to a transient "blast" of hypercoagulability. Fortunately, such

Table 11.2 Risk profile for essential thrombocytosis

Low Risk

Age < 60 *and*

No history of thrombosis *and*

Platelet count < 1,500,000/uL *and*

No cardiovascular risk factors (e.g., smoking or obesity)

Intermediate Risk

Not low or high risk

High Risk

Age ≥ 60 *or*

A history of thrombosis

Source: Tefferi A. Risk-based management in essential thrombocythemia. In: Hematology 1999: American Society of Hematology education book. Washington, DC: American Society of Hematology, 1999:172–177.

hypercoagulability affects the venous circuit, and heparin prophylaxis effectively prevents postsplenectomy thrombosis.

Regarding predicting thrombosis risk in other states of secondary thrombocytosis, a recent study examined such patients prospectively (2). Patients were divided into those with chronic or transient secondary thrombocytosis. Seven of the 25 patients with chronic and six of the 46 patients with transient thrombocytosis suffered a thrombosis. One of the seven chronic thrombocytosis patients and three of the six transient thrombocytosis patients suffered a VTE event. Among patients with thrombosis, the reticulated platelet count was much higher, leading the authors to suggest that the "platelet retic count" might predict the thrombotic risk among patients with secondary thrombocytosis.

The thrombotic risk associated with ET is more predictable and it is important to assess and intervene so that the complications of ET may be minimized. Complications most often are vasomotor symptoms and arterial thrombosis. Vasomotor symptoms, which develop in about one-third of ET patients, include headache, light-headedness, acral paresthesias, livedo reticularis, and erythromelalgia. Arterial thrombosis, such as stroke, coronary artery thrombosis, and limb ischemia, develop in about one-quarter of ET patients. Both venous thromboembolism and bleeding infrequently occur, and the risk of either of these complications is less than 1% per year. Dr. Andrew Tefferi has suggested that a simple thrombosis risk profile can be established for ET patients (Table 11.2).

The risk of thrombosis in untreated high-risk patients is about 25% at 2 years, whereas the risk of thrombosis in low-risk persons is not increased above that of age and sex matched controls (1). Low-risk ET patients suffer no additional morbidity or mortality with surgery, and the course and outcome of pregnancy are unaffected (1). In fact, low-risk patients should feel confident that their ET will not have any significant impact on their health.

Management

Secondary Thrombocytosis

Cytoreduction is not used for patients with secondary thrombocytosis. In patients who suffer symptoms of arterial thrombosis related to other conditions, routine therapy (which often includes aspirin) should be employed, but cytoreduction is not indicated. In a patient suffering thromboses whose platelet count is above 1 million/µL and who has never been evaluated for thrombocytosis, antiplatelet therapy and cytoreduction (including plateletpheresis) should be instituted and maintained until the diagnosis of secondary thrombocytosis is established.

Essential Thrombocytosis

The primary and secondary preventive management of an ET patient are identical. Every patient should receive one baby aspirin per day, for the rest of their lives, except in those extremely rare cases when bleeding is worsened by aspirin. Aspirin is particularly helpful for patients with vasomotor symptoms. High-risk patients should have their platelet count normalized, or at least reduced below 600,000/µL. Intermediate-risk patients should be considered for cytoreduction only after risk factor reduction (such as quitting smoking) fails. Women of childbearing age in the intermediate-risk category (e.g., an otherwise risk-free 25-year-old with a platelet count of 1,600,000/µL) probably should not receive cytoreduction. The management of acute thrombosis in patients with a history of ET, or in a patient who presents with thrombosis associated with an unexplained thrombocytosis, must involve *intensive rapid cytoreduction with plateletpheresis* whenever the platelet count is over 1 million/µL. When patients who are successfully cytoreduced continue to suffer symptoms of thrombosis, aspirin should be changed to clopidogrel or ticlopidine. Warfarin is only used when VTE occurs, and it is only a short-term protocol as per the routine management of VTE.

Three drugs are routinely used to reduce platelet counts in patients with ET. The treatment of choice is hydroxyurea. α2-Interferon and anagrelide are also available. Each has a distinct therapeutic index.

Hydroxyurea inhibits ribonucleotide reductase, thereby interfering with DNA synthesis. It is administered at 500 mg orally per day, with the dose escalating by increments of 500 mg (once per day or in two to three divided doses). Patients who present with very high platelet counts (>1,500,000/µL) are sometimes given 2 to 3 grams per day (loading) until the platelet count begins falling, at which time the smaller maintenance dose is started. The dose targets the platelet count, and the major dose-limiting effect is reduction of the granulocytes and red cells. Its half-life is short; without loading, the blood counts should not fall for at least 3 or more days. Patients beginning hydroxyurea should have the complete blood counts monitored twice per month until a therapeutic stable plateau in blood counts is achieved, at which time monitoring need be done only every 2 to 4 months.

Other uncommon side effects are rash, hyperpigmentation, leg ulcers, nausea, diarrhea, and hepatitis. Although hydroxyurea is a likely mutagen, there are no data indicating that it increases the risk of leukemic transformation in ET patients. Nonetheless, it should not be used injudiciously in younger patients and it should be avoided in women planning a family, or in pregnant or nursing women. It does not have an appreciable effect on fertility. Hydroxyurea is relatively inexpensive, costing about $3 per day for a 1-gram dose. When it was used to reduce platelet counts in ET patients, it resulted in a sevenfold decrease in the risk of recurrent thrombosis (3.6% versus 24% at about 3 years) (3).

α_2-Interferon is a natural leukocyte product produced for human use by genetic engineering. It causes suppression of all marrow cell lines. Its mechanism of action is pleiotropic, and the relative importance of its inhibition of various reactions directing the transcription and translation of various genes, in establishing its therapeutic index, is unknown. It is administered by subcutaneous injection. The starting dose should be low; I prefer 1 million units, three times per week. This protocol, in conjunction with regular doses of acetaminophen, minimizes the flu-like symptoms that have permanently driven many a patient away from this medicine. Over the course of 2 to 3 months, the dose should be doubled, then extended to Monday through Friday, then extended to daily doses, and finally dose-increased by 1 million units per day until a therapeutic platelet count is observed.

This program will make the α_2-interferon better tolerated, but one must still confront other common side effects including anorexia, fatigue, confusion, depression (including major psychotic depression), rashes, alopecia, and thyroiditis. Most importantly, experience with long-term use is inadequate to establish safety in young high-risk patients for whom life-long treatment is indicated. For this reason, I would not recommend its use in anyone who might need it for 5 years or more. Patients who do receive it for long periods must be monitored carefully for changes in mental status and for physical signs of a connective tissue disorder resembling scleroderma, both of which may not be reversible when the interferon is stopped. α_2-Interferon costs about $30 per day for 2 million units.

Anagrelide is a synthetic compound that inhibits platelet production, possibly due to its effect on blocking a cyclic 3′,5′-adenosine monophosphate phosphodiesterase. It also inhibits platelet aggregation. It has a short half-life and is generally dosed at 0.5 mg orally, four times a day, up to a maximal dose of 4 mg per day. It may take up to 4 weeks to effect adequate platelet reduction, which is expected in almost anyone who can tolerate it (4). The major side effect is intravascular volume expansion, and anagrelide must be used very carefully in patients with edematous states, especially congestive heart failure. Other side effects include palpitations, headache, nausea, diarrhea, and rash. Anagrelide can be used as a single agent, and is useful as an adjunct for patients whose granulocytes and/or red cell counts fall to clinically significant levels due to hydroxyurea. It is safe to decrease the dose of hydroxyurea and add anagrelide to such patients' treatment programs, as anagrelide only rarely causes anemia and probably never causes neutropenia. Currently, 2 mg of anagrelide costs about $15.

Annotated Bibliography

1. Tefferi A. Risk-based management in essential thrombocythemia. In: Hematology 1999: American Society of Hematology education book. Washington, DC: American Society of Hematology, 1999:172–177.

   A thorough, up-to-date review, including some original data about the impact of ET on pregnancy.

2. Rinder HM, Schuster JE, Rinder CS, et al. Correlation of thrombosis with increased platelet turnover in thrombocytosis. Blood 1998;91:1288–1294.

   An interesting paper for several reasons. It catalogues the types of thromboses in patients with ET and secondary thrombocytosis. Among ET patients in this study, 4 out of 9 suffered erythromelalgia and 2 out of 9 had arterial thrombosis. Among the secondary thrombocytosis patients, 7 of the 25 chronic and 6 of the 46 transient thrombocytosis patients suffered a thrombosis, the majority of which were arterial. The article also provides a window into some causes of secondary thrombocytosis: sickle cell disease, postsplenectomy, iron deficiency anemia, diabetes, rheumatoid arthritis, and malignancy. Finally, it presents data that the reticulated (RNA-containing) platelet count is much higher in all patients who have suffered thrombosis; this may be particularly useful information for deciding when to use antiplatelet therapy in those with chronic secondary thrombocytosis (patients with thrombosis showed 16.7% reticulated platelets, versus 3.1% reticulated platelets in those without thrombosis).

3. Cortelazzo S, Finazzi G, Ruggeri M, et al. Hydroxyurea for patients with essential thrombocythemia and high risk of thrombosis. New Engl J Med 1995;332:1132–1136.

   This study randomly assigned 114 patients with ET to either nothing or hydroxyurea targeted to a platelet count of below 600,000/μL. Two of the 56 treated and 14 of the 58 untreated patients suffered thromboses during a median follow-up period of 27 months.

4. Anagrelide Study Group. Anagrelide, a therapy for thrombocythemic states: experience in 577 patients. Am J Med 1992;92:69–76.

   Anagrelide is useful in reducing platelet counts. Its side effects are catalogued in this article.

12

Thrombotic Thrombocytopenic Purpura and the Hemolytic-Uremic Syndrome

Thrombotic thrombocytopenic purpura (TTP) and the hemolytic-uremic syndrome (HUS) are overlapping clinical disorders designated *thrombotic microangiopathies*. They are clinically similar because both are caused by platelet thrombus formation in the microcirculation (venules, capillaries, and arterioles) and because both can be lethal. In TTP, there are many sites of deposition, including the microcirculation of the brain, heart, spleen, kidneys, intestine, pancreas, and adrenals. In HUS, the kidneys are the major sites of platelet-mediated vaso-occlusion. TTP and HUS thereafter assume distinctive characteristics. TTP is generally an idiopathic disorder of adults, whereas HUS is generally an enterotoxin-induced disease of children. Although the pathogenesis of both TTP and HUS involves endothelial dysfunction, only in TTP is there a deficiency of a blood enzyme (designated *von Willebrand factor cleaving protease*) that breaks down unusually large (and presumed pathogenic) von Willebrand factor (vWF) multimers into smaller, more benign molecules. Finally, the natural history and outcome for TTP versus HUS are strikingly different. Untreated TTP is almost always fatal, but treatment with plasma exchange therapy cures 80% to 90% of all patients with idiopathic TTP (1,2). In contrast, HUS is only rarely lethal without or with treatment, and treatments that are effective for TTP have little impact on the natural history of HUS. The mainstay of treatment of HUS is supportive care; despite the early institution of intensive support (including hemodialysis), irreversible renal failure develops in about one-third of all HUS patients.

Clinical Features

There are less than 1000 new cases of TTP annually in the United States. There is a 2 to 1 female predominance. TTP usually is de novo and idiopathic, but there may be an association between TTP and certain underlying diseases, particularly rheumatologic diseases and acquired immunodeficiency syndrome (AIDS), and TTP can develop during the third trimester of pregnancy. There are also several drugs that have been associated with TTP, the most notorious of which is the antiplatelet agent ticlopidine (3,4).

Classic TTP presents a pentad of clinical findings: fever, microangiopathic hemolytic anemia, thrombocytopenia, neurologic signs, and renal insufficiency. This pentad is a bit misleading, as fevers are uncommon and renal failure may affect only one-half of patients, whereas abdominal pain and tenderness may be found in over one-half of all cases. The range of neurologic symptoms and signs is broad because it results from focal or multifocal ischemia of the brain; headache is not considered a significant neurologic symptom. The blood abnormalities are usually obvious, with severe anemia and thrombocytopenia, numerous circulating schistocytes and reticulocytes, negative Coombs' testing, and a serum lactate dehydrogenase (LDH) level that climbs into the thousands. The clinical course is usually treacherously rapid, and treatment must be started as soon as the diagnosis (and even the possibility of the diagnosis) of TTP appears. With effective therapy, up to 90% of all TTP cases should achieve remission, but at least 20% of those in remission will relapse. The pattern of relapse is intermittent and unpredictable, but fortunately each relapse remains treatable.

HUS is a triad of renal failure, microangiopathic hemolytic anemia, and thrombocytopenia. It is most often seen in children following a diarrheal illness: about 50% of all pediatric cases are preceded by enterocolitis. Sporadic or epidemic enterocolitides caused by toxin secreting strains of *Shigella* or *Escherichia coli* 0157:H7 are notoriously dangerous because of their association with HUS: about 15% of children suffering from enterocolitis due to *E coli* 0157:H7 will develop HUS. The toxin enters the systemic circulation and directly damages vascular endothelium. Its predilection for renal microvascular beds is presumed, but the reason for this is unknown. HUS is rare in adults, but can be associated with allogeneic stem cell transplantation, certain drugs (mitomycin, cyclosporine, and FK506 [tacrolimus]), and the postpartum state.

HUS is generally not treatable, and end-stage renal failure develops in up to one-third of all patients. Infection-associated HUS is single episode, but nondiarrheal HUS recurs in up to 15% of cases.

Differential Diagnosis

The primary diagnostic consideration in an acutely ill person with thrombocytopenia and microangiopathic hemolytic anemia is TTP versus disseminated intravascular coagulation (DIC). In every patient for whom this differential diagnosis is generated, the aPTT and PT must be examined. If they are normal, the patient has TTP and all appropriate interventions must begin immediately. If they are abnormal, the patient has DIC and treatment for its cause must begin immediately. Very rarely, a patient who has suffered severe untreated TTP will present with superimposed DIC from tissue ischemia and/or septic shock related to bowel infarction. It is probably impossible to identify TTP as the cause of the DIC that develops in this setting, and the initiation of plasma exchange therapy in this situation is often based more on a hunch than on any objective measures.

Other important diagnostic considerations include malignant hypertension, vasculitis involving the kidney, and renal allograft rejection. Each of these causes a mild microangiopathic hemolytic anemia and azotemia without dramatic thrombocytopenia or any neurologic symptoms, and the history and bedside examination are usually sufficient to establish the diagnosis.

When the possibility of TTP arises in a pregnant woman during the third trimester, one must first try to establish if the diagnosis is preeclampsia, eclampsia, or the HELLP syndrome. Preeclampsia and eclampsia are predominantly renal in origin, and hypertension, edema, and proteinuria are more prominent clinical features than are microangiopathic hemolytic anemia and thrombocytopenia. *HELLP* refers to a type of preeclampsia characterized by *h*emolytic anemia with *e*levated *l*iver enzymes and *l*ow *p*latelets. HELLP generally is a condition with mild anemia and mild thrombocytopenia. In third-trimester pregnant women who have microangiopathic hemolytic anemia and thrombocytopenia, a physician must be vigilant and prepared to use plasma exchange therapy (with or without prednisone) whenever TTP cannot be ruled out and there is clinical deterioration. A high-risk obstetrician must be involved in the care of such women, and must provide fetal monitoring and be prepared to deliver the baby (to cure preeclampsia or overt eclampsia) or perform a cesarean section (to save the infant of a woman undergoing life-saving plasma exchange for TTP).

Pathophysiology

Except for certain bacterial toxins, the cause of the thrombotic microangiopathies is not known. The model of toxin-induced endothelial cell damage has been extended to establish the theory that all thrombotic microangiopathies involve some insult to the vascular endothelium. The fact that total body irradiation (part of most stem cell therapies) and cyclosporine are recognized as causing both HUS and vascular endothelial damage is consistent with this theory. The pathological consequence of endothelial injury is the release of very large vWF multimers from the endothelial cells into the blood. Under the rheologic forces of the microcirculation, these large vWF multimers stick to platelets, cause aggregation, and form occlusive thrombi. TTP is devastating without treatment because platelet thrombi can occlude the microcirculation of virtually every organ and tissue, and it is rapidly progressive and lethal because the surface area of the affected microcirculation is immense, both relatively (as it comprises 99% of the surface area of the entire vascular tree) and absolutely (as it is roughly the size of two tennis courts). HUS is less lethal because platelets plug the renal microcirculation but do not plug elsewhere.

This vWF model of the pathogenesis of TTP and HUS is now being somewhat reorganized. This is because it needs to incorporate the discovery that most patients with TTP (both idiopathic and drug-induced) have a deficiency of a vWF-cleaving protease that breaks down the very large vWF multimers (5). This deficiency appears to be due to an antibody that blocks its activity (6). The relationship between endothelial injury and the antibody is unknown, but it provides a good explanation why large vWF multimers, which usually are not present in healthy persons, can be found in the blood of patients at the time that TTP is just starting to develop (7). The vWF-cleaving protease is not deficient in patients with HUS. This is additional evidence that the pathophysiology of HUS and TTP is different, and it may some day provide a clinical tool for establishing diagnosis and guiding therapy.

Management

TTP and HUS are true hematologic emergencies. Because it is difficult to distinguish the two clinical entities early in the course of a potentially lethal thrombotic microangiopathy, one should "treat that which is treatable," namely TTP. Figure 12.1 provides an algorithm for treatment. In addition to this approach, one must be prepared to implement intensive supportive measures, including mechanical ventilation, pressor support, and hemodialysis. Although there are some clinical data that support the idea of a "stepwise" approach to treatment using prednisone or prednisolone alone in patients with mild TTP (2), this is generally a risky approach that should be considered only for patients with mild microangiopathic hemolytic anemia and thrombocytopenia and **no other clinical manifestations**. A stepwise approach is risky because the natural history of TTP is unpredictable and because it might delay the use of standard treatment based on our current understanding that reversing the pathophysiology of TTP requires both eliminating the large vWF multimers (through plasmapheresis) and providing the vWF-cleaving protease (through plasma infusion). When plasma exchange works, relapses are minimized when the exchange program continues for 3 days after a complete remission is obtained.

The algorithm in Figure 12.1 includes substituting cryoprecipitate-poor plasma for fresh frozen plasma (FFP) during intensive plasma exchange if the clinical picture does not improve or deteriorates. Cryoprecipitate is prepared by thawing FFP at 4°C. Under this condition, the thawed liquid lacks vWF, factor VIII, fibrinogen, fibronectin, and factor XIII. When vWF is eliminated from the plasma that is infused in such patients, any pathogenic effect of the transfused FFP ("feeding the fire") is eliminated. Similarly, platelet transfusions should never be given to patients with TTP except in one circumstance: *life-threatening hemorrhage*. This is because platelet transfusions worsen the thrombotic microangiopathy and, rarely, will precipitate lethal microvascular complications.

There is no standard treatment for patients who are refractory to all exchange therapies. Several interventions could be used, including more intensive immunosuppressive therapy (with cyclophosphamide or azathioprine), vin-

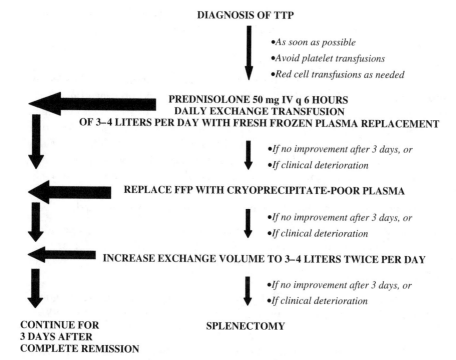

DIAGNOSIS OF TTP

- *As soon as possible*
- *Avoid platelet transfusions*
- *Red cell transfusions as needed*

PREDNISOLONE 50 mg IV q 6 HOURS
DAILY EXCHANGE TRANSFUSION
OF 3–4 LITERS PER DAY WITH FRESH FROZEN PLASMA REPLACEMENT

- *If no improvement after 3 days, or*
- *If clinical deterioration*

REPLACE FFP WITH CRYOPRECIPITATE-POOR PLASMA

- *If no improvement after 3 days, or*
- *If clinical deterioration*

INCREASE EXCHANGE VOLUME TO 3–4 LITERS TWICE PER DAY

- *If no improvement after 3 days, or*
- *If clinical deterioration*

CONTINUE FOR
3 DAYS AFTER
COMPLETE REMISSION

SPLENECTOMY

Figure 12.1.   Treatment of thrombotic thrombocytotic purpura.

cristine, or performing a splenectomy (which is preferred in our institution). Splenectomy is also useful in decreasing relapses in patients with chronic relapsing TTP (8).

Children who have infection-associated HUS should *not* receive antibacterial therapy. Despite the logic that eradicating toxin producing bacteria should work, there is ample clinical evidence that it does not work. In fact, antibiotic treatment directed at *E coli* 0157 : H7 increases the risk that HUS will develop (9).

Annotated Bibliography

1. Rock GA, Shumak KH, Buskard NA, et al. Comparison of plasma exchange with plasma infusion in the treatment of thrombotic thrombocytopenic purpura. The Canadian Apheresis Study Group. New Engl J Med 1991;325:393–397.

   In this study 102 TTP patients were randomized to receive either plasma exchange or plasma infusion. After 7 days of therapy 24 of 51 patients receiving plasma exchange, and 13 of 51 receiving plasma infusion, had a hematologic response. Eleven of the 51 patients who received a plasma exchange and 19 of the 51 who received plasma infusions died.

2. Bell WR, Hayden GB, Ness PM, Kickler TS. Improved survival in thrombotic thrombocytopenic purpura–hemolytic uremic syndrome. New Engl J Med 1991;325:398–403.

   This is a descriptive analysis of 108 patients treated at Johns Hopkins University Hospital from 1979 through 1990. Thirty patients were labeled as suffering from "mild" TTP/HUS (minimal symptoms and no central nervous symptoms except headache). All of these patients were treated with 200 mg prednisone per day, and 28 of the 30 survived, with only two relapses among the survivors. In the 78 patients who had less mild TTP/HUS, 200 mg per day prednisone was administered, plus plasma exchange. There was no standard program of plasma exchange, which was generally undertaken daily until a response was observed. Eleven of the 78 patients were cured with exchange therapy; however, 67 of the 78 relapsed, and 7 of these patients died.

3. Tsai HM, Rice LR, Sarode R, et al. Antibody inhibitors to von Willebrand factor metalloproteinase and increased binding of von Willebrand factor to platelets in ticlopidine-associated thrombotic thrombocytopenic purpura. Ann Intern Med 2000;132:794–799.

   Seven patients who developed TTP 2 to 7 weeks after beginning ticlopidine were studied. All had an IgG antibody that inhibited the activity of the vWF-cleaving protease.

4. Bennet CL, Connors JM, Carwile JM, et al. Thrombotic thrombocytopenic purpura associated with clopidogrel. New Engl J Med 2000;342:1773–1777.

   Clopidogrel causes TTP. Its estimated incidence is about 1 per 300,000 users. The estimated incidence of ticlopidine-related TTP is about 1 per 3000 cases.

5. Furlan M, Robles R, Galbusera M, et al. Von Willebrand factor–cleaving protease in thrombotic thrombocytopenic purpura and the hemolytic-uremic syndrome. New Engl J Med 1998;339:1578–1584.

   The assay for vWF cleaving protease is cumbersome: high concentrations of urea are required to unfold the enzyme into an active conformation. How can this relate to physiological activity? It may be that shearing forces generated by flowing blood affect the protease just as urea affects it: shear stress opens it up into an active conformation like the wind unfurls a sail. The vWF cleaving protease was absent in 24 of 24 patients with acquired TTP and was normal in 11 of 13 patients with HUS.

6. Tsai H-M, Lian E. Antibodies to von Willebrand factor–cleaving protease in acute thrombotic thrombocytopenic purpura. New Engl J Med 1998;339:1585–1594.

   Plasma from 37 patients with acute TTP was deficient in the protease that cleaves large vWF multimers; 67% of the plasma samples had an IgG antibody that inhibited the proteolytic activity of the vWF cleaving protease.

7. Moake JL. Moschcowitz, multimers, and metalloprotease. New Engl J Med 1998;339:1629–1631.

A brief review of TTP that blends the author's lifelong devotion to the vWF hypothesis with the recent breakthrough discovery of an acquired enzyme deficiency that could account for the presence of pathological vWF multimers in patients with TTP.

8. Crowther MA, Heddle N, Hayward C, et al. Splenectomy done during hematologic remission to prevent relapse in patients with thrombotic thrombocytopenic purpura. Ann Intern Med 1996;125:294–296.

This is a consecutive case series of six patients with chronic relapsing TTP who underwent therapeutic splenectomy while in a hematologic remission. There was an average of about one relapse per year before splenectomy, and about one relapse per 8 years after splenectomy.

9. Wong CS, Jelacic S, Habeeb RL, et al. The risk of hemolytic-uremic syndrome after antibiotic treatment of *Escherichia coli* 0157:H7 infections. New Engl J Med 2000;342:1930–1936.

This is an informative prospective evaluation of 71 children who had culture-positive infection. Almost every child had bloody diarrhea and vomiting, and 10 of the children developed HUS. None of these children (actually none of the 71 children) died. Four patients suffered oligoanuric renal failure. The relative risk of developing HUS was almost 18 for children who received trimethoprim-sulfamethoxazole and 13 for those who received a β-lactam antibiotic.

13

An Overview of Hemorrhagic Disorders and Their Treatment

Bleeding is always a sign that something is wrong somewhere in Virchow's triad. It might simply reflect an obvious structural problem, like a bleeding duodenal ulcer or hemopleuropericardium from a loose coronary artery bypass graft. Or it might reflect a subtle but potentially dangerous problem with a plasma coagulation protein, like the congenital deficiency of factor XI. A daily challenge faced by medical consultants who work closely with surgeons is to rank the importance of several abnormalities that are present simultaneously during the perioperative period in bleeding patients. This task must be more than a scholarly exercise, and time may not allow one to objectify or rule out every interesting possibility that one discovers—as, for example, when one must explore the differential diagnosis of a patient whose blood pressure and hemoglobin concentration are dropping after coming off cardiopulmonary bypass.

The next several chapters present information that allows one to approach the diagnosis and treatment of bleeding problems rationally. However, one must never delay potentially life-saving treatment because of uncertainty about the pathophysiology of a bleeding problem. Chances are good that if the operating surgeon wants platelets, fresh frozen plasma, and cryoprecipitate for a patient who is exsanguinating, that patient will benefit from these blood products— even if the platelet count is reasonable, the prothrombin time is barely abnormal, and a thrombin time measurement hasn't been ordered. Our job is to optimize hemostasis and minimize bleeding, while maximizing the therapeutic index of specific interventions. We must therefore sometimes "shotgun" first, and resolve diagnoses second: *primum non nocere*.

The Bedside Exam

Bleeding is of two varieties, each of which provides diagnostic information.

Superficial bleeding is caused by abnormalities of the vessel wall or platelets. Superficial bleeding in the skin results in petechiae and ecchymoses. Superficial bleeding also involves mucosal surfaces resulting in conjunctival bleeding, nose bleeding, gum bleeding, urinary bleeding, and rectal bleeding. In the United States, superficial bleeding is most often caused by thrombocytopenia (see Chapter 14), but mild deficiency of von Willebrand factor (vWF)—von Willebrand disease—leading to mild superficial bleeding is very common (see Chapter 16). Of note, von Willebrand disease can also lead to hemophilia-type bleeding (as discussed below) because vWF is the carrier protein for factor VIII. The character of the superficial hemorrhage may provide prognostic significance: "wet purpura" is a glistening dark submucosal collection of red cells on the palate or in the oropharynx that reflects severe dysfunction of platelet–vessel wall interactions. The presence of wet purpura in a patient with thrombocytopenia indicates that immediate treatment is required. Similarly, a fresh "shower" of petechiae in a patient with underproduction thrombocytopenia is usually an indication for platelet transfusions. Although spontaneous intracranial bleeding is rare, the presence of wet purpura and/or petechial showers should be considered a harbinger of severe bleeding and platelet transfusions should be administered as rapidly as possible.

The second variety of bleeding is deep bleeding due to deficiency or dysfunction of the coagulation proteins. Persons suffering from hemophilia due to congenital factor VIII or factor IX deficiency will experience spontaneous bleeding into the joints (hemarthrosis), into muscles, into viscera, and into the soft tissues of the retroperitoneum. Spontaneous intracranial hemorrhage is rare, but the most trivial trauma (dismissed without thought in a healthy person) can cause intracranial bleeding in a patient with severe hemophilia.

Bleeding that doesn't occur spontaneously but develops after provocation (like surgery or trauma) is typical of factor XI deficiency, which is common in Ashkenazi Jews. Similarly, congenital deficiency of factor XIII (fibrin-stabilizing factor), which is very rare, is associated with bleeding after provocation, delayed bleeding, and poor wound healing. Of note, factor XIII deficiency is, for unknown reasons, associated with spontaneous intracranial bleeding in up to one-quarter of all affected persons.

Laboratory Testing

Chapter 2 describes the laboratory tests used to evaluate a bleeding patient. Table 2.1 presents a hierarchical series of studies to evaluate a coagulation factor disorder, with each tier after first tier testing (the **PT, aPTT,** and **thrombin time**) narrowing the diagnostic focus. The second tier includes **mixing studies** (to evaluate an abnormal PT and/or aPTT) to identify an inhibitor or a coagulation factor deficiency; **D-dimer assay** to evaluate for disseminated intravascular coagulation (DIC) or hyperfibrinolysis; and the **reptilase time** to determine if the coagulopathy is due to the presence of systemic heparin or heparin contaminating the blood draw. The third tier includes measuring **factor levels** (to specify and quantify the coagulation protein deficiency); and the **vWF antigen level** and **ristocetin cofactor activity** (to establish the presence and type of von Willebrand disease). Fourth tier testing includes **urea lysis** (to test for the stability of fibrin cross-linked by factor XIII); **vWF multimers** (to establish type II von Willebrand disease); and tests for deficiencies of antifibrinolytic proteins such as α_2 **anti-plasmin level.**

Fewer tests are available for evaluating superficial bleeding due to abnormalities of platelet-endothelial interactions. The platelet count is the first tier test. When it is decreased unexpectedly in an asymptomatic person, one must double-check that it isn't **pseudothrombocytopenia** (see Chapter 14). When it is normal in a patient with superficial bleeding, one moves to second tier testing with a **bleeding time** (used to investigate qualitative platelet problems—see Chapter 15; von Willebrand disease—see Chapter 16; and vascular purpura, such as Cushing's disease or scurvy). **Platelet aggregation** can be used simultaneously or subsequent to the bleeding time to evaluate for von Willebrand disease, or to identify a rare disorder of deficient storage granules, dysfunctional platelet signaling pathways, or abnormal surface glycoprotein receptors. Impaired storage pools or defective signaling might lead to impaired platelet secretion, which is evaluated in special laboratories equipped either with a **lumi-aggregometer**, which measures released adenosine triphosphate (ATP) using luciferase luminescence, or with a radiation safety license so that the **release of** $[^{14}C]$ **serotonin** taken up by platelet dense granules may be measured. Finally, storage pool diseases and some inherited diseases of platelets result in morphologic changes that are identified by **electron microscopy.**

Principles of Replacement Therapy

Blood products are administered to patients who are sick because their blood is missing something. In bleeding disorders, the deficiency could result from either decreased quantity of a coagulation factor or decreased circulating platelets. There also could be deficient activity because of a qualitative problem or because there is a circulating inhibitor. In all of these cases, the disease is treated by attempting to restore the missing blood component. Blood products are therefore drugs, and their regulation and use are driven by the therapeutic index: the balance between efficacy and toxicity.

Most blood products are derived from human donors and, despite extensive donor screening and post-donation blood testing, all blood products derived from human donors carry the risk of transmitting an infectious disease. To minimize this risk, blood products undergo a variety of purification steps, including

- Heating above 60°C to inactivate human immunodeficiency virus (HIV)
- Wet heating above 80°C to inactivate hepatitis B virus (HBV), hepatitis C virus (HCV), and hepatitis A (HAV)
- Pasteurization to inactivate HIV, HBV, and HCV
- Solvent/detergent extraction to inactivate HIV, HBV, and HCV (but not HAV)
- Ultrafiltration with elution in sodium thiocyanate to inactivate HIV, HBV, and HCV
- Photodecontamination to eliminate all viruses

Table 13.1 Viral transmission risk per unit of blood product transfused

VIRUS	RISK
Human immunodeficiency virus (HIV)	2/1,000,000
Hepatitis B virus (HBV)	16/1,000,000
Hepatitis C virus (HCV)	10/1,000,000
Human T-cell leukemia virus 1 (HTLV)	2/1,000,000[a]

[a] For cellular elements only; no risk with plasma-derived products.

Despite using one or more of these processes, there is a measurable risk of blood product transmission of a viral infection. Platelets are usually transfused from a bag pooled from 6 to 10 donors (random donor platelets); a replacement dose of cryoprecipitate requires many donors; and purified coagulation factors are derived from literally thousands of donors. Table 13.1 gives the risk per unit transfused (1).

The data in Table 13.1 are already 5 years old, and improvements in virus inactivation have continued, making processed blood even safer and leaving most purified human products and recombinant coagulation factors with an almost infinitesimally small risk. Nonetheless, it is essential to keep track of the viral transmission data for whatever blood product one is considering using, and to factor this information judiciously into the decision to use it.

Annotated Bibliography

1. Schrieber GB, Busch MP, Kleinman SH, Korelitz JJ. The risk of transfusion-transmitted viral infections. N Engl J Med 1996;334:1685–1690.

   As stated in this study, "The risk of transmitting HIV, HTLV, HCV and HBV is very small, and new screening tests will reduce the risk even further." How small? Among donors who passed all screening tests, the risks of a contaminated donation are as follows: HIV, 1 in 493,000; human T-cell leukemia virus (HTLV), 1 in 641,000; HCV, 1 in 103,000; and HBV, 1/63,000. The aggregate risk is 1 in 34,000.

14

Thrombocytopenia

Thrombocytopenia is due to destruction, sequestration, underproduction, or dilution of blood platelets. Destruction is either immune or nonimmune. Sequestration is due to hypersplenism. Underproduction is most often due to myelosuppressive chemotherapy. Dilution is due to massive intravascular loading by fluid replacement and/or red cell transfusions. Destruction and sequestration are often accompanied by marrow megakaryocyte hyperplasia and the release of young ("giant") platelets into the blood. Underproduction is usually represented by a paucity of marrow megakaryocytes. Underproduction can also result from "ineffective megakaryocytopoiesis," and it is interesting to note that immune thrombocytopenias (ITPs) frequently demonstrate impaired platelet production along with precursor cell hyperplasia.

Both bleeding risk and bleeding time vary with the type of thrombocytopenia (1). Figure 14.1 shows that in underproduction (and dilutional) thrombocytopenia there is a linear inverse relationship between the platelet count and the bleeding time such that all patients with counts below 10,000/µL have bleeding times that are greatly elevated (e.g., over 30 minutes) and will likely have some type of superficial bleeding. In contrast, the bleeding time is usually normal or only slightly elevated in ITP, whereas von Willebrand disease (vWD) is associated with elevated bleeding times despite normal platelet counts. Similarly, uremia and other acquired or inherited disorders of platelet function result in elevated bleeding times despite the blood platelet counts being normal. (See Chapters 15 and 16.)

Regulation of Platelet Production

The regulation of blood platelet counts involves several growth factors that stimulate megakaryocyte proliferation and maturation (2). The most important is thrombopoietin, but interleukin-3, IL-6, IL-11, and other molecules are also involved (2). In fact, IL-11 is the only megakaryocyte growth factor that is approved by the U.S. Food and Drug Administration for use in attenuating chemotherapy-induced thrombocytopenia (see below). The regulation of blood platelet counts involves 1) the fairly steady production of thrombopoietin (TPO)

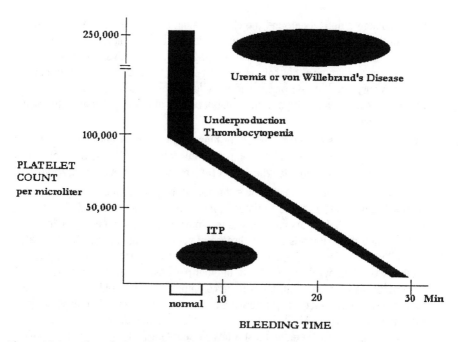

Figure 14.1. The relationship between bleeding time and platelet count.

by the liver, 2) a sensor (the circulating platelets), and 3) a responder (the megakaryocyte). Platelets have TPO receptors and they bind TPO in the blood. When platelet counts are low, there is decreased TPO binding leading to increased levels of free TPO, and this drives marrow megakaryocytopoiesis and the release of platelets. When platelet counts are normal, levels of free TPO decrease and platelet production decreases. Blood TPO levels in response to both physiological and pathological forces vary greatly, however, and the only state of absolute TPO deficiency likely to be identified (and treated effectively by TPO administration) is found in some liver transplant recipients.

Clinical Aspects of ITP

ITP is a clinical diagnosis. It presents typically with a low platelet count accompanied by preserved hemoglobin concentration and leukocyte count. It may be idiopathic, associated with a drug, or secondary to a lymphoproliferative disorder, a connective tissue disorder, or (particularly in children) an infection. The low platelet count may be discovered incidentally, or it may be measured because a patient has complained of a petechial rash, easy bruising, and/or mucosal bleeding. Only three tests are used to evaluate a patient for ITP.

- *Blood Smear.* The blood smear should be examined to rule out *pseudothrombocytopenia* due to platelet clumping while EDTA (purple top) or citrate (blue top) anticoagulated blood sits around the clinical hematology lab before analysis. These calcium-binding anticoagulants will leach calcium out of the platelet cytosol and out of cytosolic calcium storage pools, resulting in platelet activation causing aggregation or *clumping* that can be seen on smear. Whenever pseudothrombocy-topenia is suspected, based on unexpectedly low platelets and clumping on smear, it is confirmed by measuring a normal platelet count in blood anticoagulated with heparin (green top tube).

- *HIV Testing.* Patients should be tested for human immunodeficiency virus (HIV) because ITP in adults commonly accompanies this infection. ITP has been observed in up to 10% of AIDS patients who have CD4 lymphocyte counts below 250/μL.

- *Bone Marrow Evaluation.* Patients over the age of 60 years should have a bone marrow evaluation to rule out a primary bone marrow disease, particularly myelodysplasia (3). The rationale for this recommendation is solid epidemiologic data showing that ITP tends to be a disease of young people (usually 20–40 years old) and women (3 : 1 predominance). There are no solid data about the relative frequency of myelodysplasia versus ITP in older persons, but in our institution myelodysplasia is at least four times more common than ITP in older men. The ITP bone marrow shows megakaryocyte hyperplasia with fairly normal erythropoiesis and granulocytopoiesis. Myelodysplasia is often a trilineage disorder associated with small megakaryocytes containing just a few nuclear lobes, and both quantitatively and qualitatively (*morphologically*) abnormal myeloid and erythroid development.

Treatments for ITP

ITP treatment probably should be given whenever the platelet count is below 30,000/μL, even when the patient is not bleeding (3). Treatment always begins with corticosteroid administration. If a patient is taking a drug that causes ITP, that drug should be stopped immediately. If the patient is infected with HIV and it is a new diagnosis, the patient should have antiretroviral therapy instituted immediately if the viral load is greater than 20,000/mL or if the CD4 count is below 350/μL. If acquired immunodeficiency syndrome (AIDS) is an old diagnosis, the efficacy of antiretroviral therapy should be assessed and the drug program modified to optimize the antiviral response and immune reconstitution.

The treatment of ITP with bleeding is a hematologic emergency. Patients should be started on prednisone (2 mg/kg) plus intravenous immunoglobulin (IVIG), 1 gm/kg every day for 1 to 2 days. If the bleeding is life threatening, patients should also receive platelet transfusions. Ideally, platelets should be administered after the first dose of IVIG. If platelets are used immediately they should be given in very large doses (such as 8 units of random donor platelets given three times over 2 hours). This will enhance survival and increase the platelet response, probably because the first half of the total transfused platelets temporarily binds up the antibody.

The treatment of adults with ITP, including HIV-associated ITP (4), who are not bleeding is diagrammed in Figure 14.2. Pediatric ITP is usually ephemeral

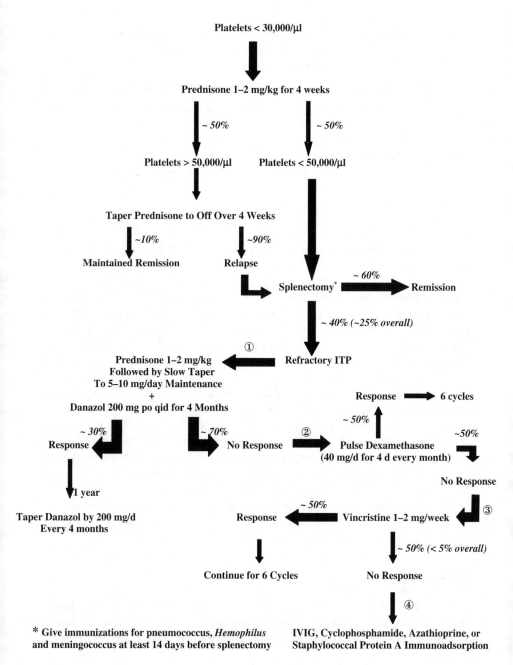

Figure 14.2.   Treatment of immune thrombocytopenias without bleeding.

Table 14.1   A comparison of intravenous immunoglobulin and anti-D antiserum for immune thrombocytopenias

IVIG (1 g/kg)	ANTI-D ANTISERUM (50 μg/kg)
2–3 liters infusion volume	15–30 mL infusion volume
Administer every 3 to 4 weeks	Administer every 1 to 3 weeks
90% respond	80% respond
$3000.00/course	$2000.00/course
Causes fevers, chills, hypotension	Causes red cell hemolysis

and follows various nonspecific viral infections. Children with low platelet counts should receive treatment with prednisone (1 mg/kg), and if there is recurrence following the steroid tapering, nonsurgical interventions should be used while waiting for the disease to run its course (usually less than 6 months). The two best-characterized treatments to use in this setting are IVIG and anti-D antiserum (WinRho SD). Both work by binding to immunoglobulin Fc receptors on splenic macrophages (IVIG directly, and anti-D attached to Rh-positive red cells), thereby blocking the destruction of antibody-coated platelets. IVIG works in splenectomized patients of any blood type, while anti-D antiserum works best in patients with a spleen and only if they have Rh-positive red cells (Table 14.1). Both IVIG and anti-D antiserum can also be used in adults with chronic ITP, although they are expensive and only work transiently.

Treatment of chronic ITP that persists after splenectomy, and for patients who refuse splenectomy and relapse after prednisone taper, is individualized. As listed below, one can use IVIG (or anti-D antiserum), immunosuppression (azathioprine, cyclophosphamide—which may be particularly useful in lupus-associated ITP [5]), or combination chemotherapy (6).

When desperation is at its apogee, one might consider splenic irradiation (7) or immunoadsorption of the offending antibody by passing small volumes of whole blood over a staphylococcal protein A column (8).

ITP During Pregnancy

There are three issues to consider in sequence when faced with a falling platelet count in a pregnant woman: establish the etiology and prognosis for the mother, optimize the pregnancy's outcome, and establish the impact of maternal thrombocytopenia on the health of the neonate.

The first issue is the cause of the condition and the prognosis for the mother. Platelet counts fall below 150,000/μL in about 7% of pregnant women (9). Among pregnant women whose platelet counts fall below this lower limit of normal, almost 75% will prove to have incidental or benign thrombocytopenia; about 21% have thrombocytopenia due to a pregnancy-related hypertensive disorder; and about 4% have ITP. No special studies are indicated or available to establish the diagnosis of ITP in pregnant women, so it remains a clinical diagnosis (3). Perhaps more importantly, no treatment for low platelets is indicated until the count falls below 50,000/µL *regardless of the cause.* And almost all women whose platelets fall to such levels *do not have incidental thrombocytopenia.* The platelet count remains above this level in almost every patient with incidental thrombocytopenia, which is defined as pregnancy-associated thrombocytopenia that returns to normal within a few days of delivery.

When the platelet count falls in a pregnant woman who has chronic ITP, a history of pregnancy-associated ITP, or a new diagnosis of ITP, the platelet count threshold for treatment increases as the pregnancy proceeds: *first trimester,* 20,000/µL; *second/third trimester,* 30,000/µL; *delivery,* 50,000/µL. ITP treatment aimed at raising the platelet count above 50,000/µL is indicated for bleeding at any time during pregnancy. Vaginal delivery is as safe as cesarean section *for both the mother and the infant* as long as the platelets are above 50,000/µL.

The second issue is ITP treatment that optimizes the outcome for the pregnancy (i.e., for both the mother and the fetus). It must be emphasized that there is no correlation between maternal and fetal platelet counts, and treating the mother has no effect on the platelet count of the newborn. A history of maternal ITP with previous delivery of a thrombocytopenic infant is the only predictor for low fetal platelet counts, and it is a weak predictor. Both IVIG and prednisone are safe and effective treatments for pregnancy-associated ITP. When neither of these interventions works and maternal risk is high because there is bleeding and the platelet count is below 10,000/µL, splenectomy can be done during the second trimester.

At the time of delivery, the maternal platelet count affects certain specific interventions. Epidural injections should be given only when platelet counts are above 50,000/µL. If the fetal platelet count is not known (as is often the situation), either cesarean section or vaginal delivery can still be done when the maternal platelet count is below 50,000/µL as long as certain contingencies are met. If platelets are over 30,000/µL and there is no bleeding, nothing needs to be done except to ensure that platelets are available for transfusion should excessive bleeding develop. Prophylactic platelet transfusions are indicated when platelets are less than 30,000/µL and the patient is having a cesarean section. They are also indicated when the platelets are below 30,000/µL, the woman has mucosal bleeding, and a vaginal delivery is planned.

The third issue is the impact of maternal thrombocytopenia on the health of the neonate. As described above, there is no relationship between a mother's and her baby's platelet counts. In fact, the risk of significant thrombocytopenia in a newborn whose mother has ITP or a history of ITP (with normal platelet counts during the pregnancy) is surprisingly small. About one-half of these newborns have decreased platelets, but only about 15% have platelet counts below 50,000/µL, and in one study none had counts below 20,000/µL (9). Similarly, the risk of intracranial hemorrhage—the major intrauterine and delivery complication—among babies with platelet counts 20,000–50,000/µL born of women with ITP was zero (9).

Because safe and reliable intrauterine platelet counts are not generally available, it is perfectly reasonable to deliver the infant as described above; one would then check the platelet count of the newborn, and initiate appropriate treatment as needed postnatally. Only when there is a history of prior clinically significant severe neonatal thrombocytopenia of any source (but particularly alloimmune thrombocytopenia) should fetal measurements be done. Fetal platelet counts should be obtained by umbilical cord sampling. This form of measurement is accurate, but is associated with 1% to 2% fetal loss. Fetal scalp vein sampling is unreliable (discordant with baby's platelet count 50% of the time) and should not be done. Cord blood sampling should only be done if it influences the management of parturition. This is not clear-cut at all, however— there is evidence that the mode of delivery doesn't affect neonate outcome even in babies whose platelets are below 50,000/µL. The American Society of Hematology advises cesarean section *only* for a fetus with ITP whose cord blood sample reveals that the platelets are below 20,000/µL.

Alloimmune Thrombocytopenia

The condition that is most threatening to the health of a fetus is alloimmune thrombocytopenia, which occurs when there is a mismatch of platelet surface antigenic proteins between the fetus and the mother. This is most commonly due to a PL^{A1} and PL^{A2} mismatch; among whites there is a 0.85 and 0.15 gene frequency, respectively. The PL^{A2} polymorphism is due to a leucine to proline substitution at position 33 in the fibrinogen receptor glycoprotein (Gp) IIIa. This change affects the structure of GpIIIa, creating a new epitope. When homozygosity for PL^{A2} occurs in a fetus ($0.15 \times 0.15 = 0.0225$, ~ 2% of all births among whites), a maternal antibody response is stimulated; the antibody crosses the placenta, and the fetus suffers thrombocytopenia very early in gestation. Thrombocytopenia is absent in mothers, but they develop life-long sensitization to the PL^{A2} epitope, and fetal thrombocytopenia tends to be worse with subsequent affected pregnancies.

The natural history of this condition is bad, and at least 25% of affected and untreated fetuses develop intracranial hemorrhage. When the diagnosis is known (usually after the birth of an affected baby), fetal platelet counts are monitored during subsequent pregnancies by umbilical cord vein sampling, usually first performed at 20 weeks.

Babies born with alloimmune thrombocytopenia usually show petechiae. They are treated with transfusion of platelets harvested by plateletpheresis from the mother, washed free of antibody-containing plasma and gamma irradiated. When alloimmune thrombocytopenia is diagnosed antenatally (based on history and umbilical vein blood sampling), treatment is indicated. The first line of treatment is giving maternal IVIG (1 gm/kg/week) for 4 to 5 weeks, followed by repeat umbilical vein sampling. This treatment results in a 74% response rate, and when it works it should be continued until delivery. If IVIG does not work, a fetal transfusion of platelets, prepared as described above, is administered at weekly intervals.

Alloimmune thrombocytopenia also causes an unusual syndrome in adults designated *posttransfusion purpura*. This is a rare but dangerous complication of transfusion (of any blood product) that typically occurs in multiparous PL^{A1}-negative women a week after they receive their first transfusion. Platelet counts are almost always below 10,000/μL, bleeding is common, and 10% of those untreated will suffer an intracranial hemorrhage. It is probably caused by a potent anti-PL^{A1} antibody present in the transfusion recipient's plasma that forms immune complexes with PL^{A1}-positive platelet fragments present in the transfused blood. These immune complexes adsorb onto the recipient's platelets and effect their destruction. Treatment should begin with prednisone *plus* IVIG, which works in the majority of cases. If IVIG fails, plasma exchange will salvage the patient. Platelet transfusions can worsen the syndrome and are relatively contraindicated. Platelet counts always recover within a month.

Drug-Induced Thrombocytopenia

The diagnosis of drug-induced thrombocytopenia is established entirely through empiricism (10). There are four empirical facts that one can apply, and the first three are safely and routinely obtained.

1. Thrombocytopenia is temporally related to starting the drug.
2. No other cause of thrombocytopenia is apparent.
3. Platelet counts recover after stopping the drug.
4. Thrombocytopenia returns when the patient is rechallenged with the drug.

There are long lists of such drug culprits based on these criteria (Table 14.2). It is generally acknowledged that any drug can be associated with thrombocytopenia, and any patient who satisfies the first two criteria listed above should have the diagnosis established by monitoring platelet counts after the drug is stopped.

How long should one wait before abandoning this diagnosis? No one really knows, but it is reasonable to wait several months for platelet counts to recover before dismissing the diagnosis of drug-induced thrombocytopenia (the half-life for an inhibitory IgG antibody is about 21 days). Except for heparin-induced thrombocytopenia, there are no laboratory tests helpful for establishing the diagnosis of drug-induced thrombocytopenia.

The mechanisms of drug-induced thrombocytopenia are marrow suppression and/or immune-mediated destruction. Table 14.2 lists in rank order the best-established culprits, with the mechanism by which they cause thrombocytopenia. Whenever drug-induced thrombocytopenia is suspected in a patient who has profoundly low platelets and bleeding, routine ITP therapy should be started. With the single exception of heparin, which will be dealt with separately in the next section, those patients with immune-mediated drug-induced thrombocytopenia almost always respond to drug withdrawal plus prednisone and/or IVIG.

Table 14.2   Mechanisms of drug-induced thrombocytopenia

DRUG	MARROW	ANTIBODY
Heparin	−	+
Ethanol	+	−
Quinidine	−	+
Quinine	−	+
TMP-Sulfa	+	+
Gold	+	+
Procainamide	−	+
Methyldopa	−	+
Carbamazepine	+	−
Hydrochlorothiazide	−	+
Penicillins	−	+
Valproic acid	+	+

Note: For a complete list see George JN, Raskob GE, Shah SR, et al. Drug-induced thrombocytopenia; a systematic review of published case reports. Ann Intern Med 1998;129:886–890.

Heparin-Induced Thrombocytopenia

Heparin-induced thrombocytopenia (HIT) is defined by a decrease in platelet count by 50%, or a decrease below 100,000/μL, in a patient receiving heparin. This occurs in 1% to 2% of all patients who receive heparin. HIT develops in all settings in which heparin is used, and can develop with heparin of any source, fraction, dosage, and route of administration. It typically occurs 4 to 7 days after heparin is started, but is more rapid in onset and of increased magnitude in patients who have received past doses of heparin (11). HIT never develops 14 or more days after heparin is stopped. The risk of HIT is lower with low-molecular-weight heparin and higher with bovine preparations of unfractionated heparin.

The only special laboratory test helpful in diagnosing immune-mediated thrombocytopenia is a test for heparin-dependent platelet antibodies. There are two tests routinely used: activity tests and antigen tests.

The best activity test is set up by incubating the patient's platelet-poor plasma with material that binds all heparin in the specimen and by incubating washed normal donor platelets with radiolabeled serotonin, which is taken up into the platelets' dense granules. The washed platelets are mixed with the patient's plasma, and heparin (ideally from the same lot that the patient received) is added back. A positive response is the release of radiolabeled serotonin at doses of heparin less than 0.5 U/mL. This test is positive in 90% of HIT cases and in virtually no other types of thrombocytopenia.

The other activity test produces more false-negative results. It is more often employed because it does not entail the use of radioactive material. The setup is identical to above, except that no serotonin is added and the response measured is platelet aggregation. This test is only 60% sensitive.

In addition to these functional tests for heparin-associated antibodies, there are several solid-phase immunoassays on the market that identify antibodies that bind to a complex of heparin and platelet factor 4 (PF4). The current understanding of the pathophysiology of HIT points to PF4 as the target epitope on platelets. PF4 is an alpha granule protein that is expressed following platelet activation. PF4 binds to heparin and neutralizes its antithrombotic activity. Most cases of HIT defined by clinical criteria (50% reduction of platelet count) are associated with high-titer antibodies to heparin/PF4 fixed onto an ELISA plate. The clinical use of ELISA methods as a screening tool or as a tool that directs specific interventions is still a bit hazy, as many patients who receive unfractionated or fractionated heparin without evidence of HIT or thrombosis show a positive antibody response in these types of heparin antibody assays.

The management of HIT is straightforward. *Every patient receiving heparin whose platelets fall by 50% or below 100,000/µL must have all heparin preparations stopped.* Heparin is stopped so that the patient's risk for HIT with thrombosis (HITT) is eliminated. HITT occurs in up to 10% of all cases of HIT. It is a dangerous syndrome of thrombosis developing in any venous or arterial circuit, but particularly affecting large arteries damaged by chronic atherosclerosis. When it goes unrecognized it can be fatal. The pathogenesis of HITT is uncertain, but appears to involve both intravascular platelet aggregation and the stimulation of vascular endothelial procoagulant activity. The treatment of HITT is not predictably efficacious, so there is a great need to prevent HITT by *stopping heparin.*

When patients taken off heparin require immediate anticoagulation, they should receive another antithrombin anticoagulant. The two that are currently available in the United States are hirudin and argatroban. Hirudin or argatroban should also be substituted for heparin in all patients with a prior episode of HIT who require subsequent anticoagulation, except patients undergoing open heart surgery 3 months after the discontinuation of heparin (see below). The most common situations where this might come up are anticoagulation for DVT, pulmonary embolism, unstable angina, or recent onset atrial fibrillation.

Hirudin is a recombinant leech protein that binds to thrombin and blocks its catalytic activity. Argatroban is a small synthetic thrombin-binding molecule derived from L-arginine. Both are FDA approved for use in HIT without or with thrombosis. They are used similarly to heparin: their anticoagulant activity is monitored by the aPTT (Table 14.3), and warfarin should be administered routinely with careful aPTT monitoring.

The treatment of HITT is a medical emergency. HITT is not usually associated with a deficiency of hemostasis, so its treatment tends to be an indelicate and rapid attempt to maximize anticoagulation. The medical management includes full anticoagulation with hirudin or argatroban, and daily aspirin. Surgical consultation should be obtained immediately, and surgical thrombectomy be performed for impending limb infarction. Coronary ischemia or infarction should be treated with a slant toward invasive interventions and a slant away

Table 14.3   Anticoagulation therapy used when a patient has heparin-induced thrombocytopenia

HIRUDIN DOSING	ARGATROBAN DOSING
0.4 mg/kg bolus	2 µg/kg/min initial dose
0.15 mg/kg/hour infusion	Titrate to maintain aPTT 1.5–25 × control
Monitor aPTT 4 hours after starting and then at least daily (target aPTT is 1.5–2.5 × control)	Steady state achieved in 2 to 3 hours
Reduce dose by 50% when creatinine is >1.5 dL	Reduce dose to 0.5 µg/kg/min when there is hepatic impairment

from thrombolysis. Thrombolytic therapy is fairly untested in HITT; for a patient with HITT suffering an acute ischemic stroke or MI being treated by tPA, hirudin may be the preferred agent when used at an infusion rate decreased to 0.1 mg/kg per hour.

Another challenge presented by the HIT phenomenon is cardiopulmonary bypass. A patient with a history of HIT who has been off heparin for 3 months or longer can receive heparin anticoagulation during the pump run, but *only during cardiopulmonary bypass* (11). In a patient who had heparin-dependent antiplatelet antibodies in the past, it is prudent to demonstrate their absence before heparin is used for cardiopulmonary bypass, although in almost every patient with HIT who was left off heparin for at least 3 months the antibody activity is absent or very low (11). No additional heparin of any sort should be administered at any time following the procedure.

In a patient with active HIT who must have cardiac surgery requiring extracorporeal circulation, one must work closely with the surgeons, pump nurse, and anesthesiologists to develop a plan for anticoagulation. There are no standard interventions, but there is some experience using hirudin, particularly in Europe. If hirudin is to be used, the dosing program needs to be individualized, and fairly intensive aPTT monitoring must be planned to optimize the dosage. In a single experience from our institution, all preparations flew out the window as soon as the pump run started and the activated clotting time (ACT), believed to be the only reliable measure by the anesthesiologists, was below target! The outcome was fine, but achieving the target ACT resulted in an aPTT that was sky high for 24 hours. A hirudin overdose associated with bleeding can be treated with fresh frozen plasma.

Underproduction Thrombocytopenia

Most thrombocytopenias are caused by bone marrow disorders. The most common disorder is iatrogenic: chemotherapy-induced. In addition there are hypoplastic syndromes (aplastic anemia), dysplastic syndromes (myelodysplasia), infiltrative disorders (leukemias, lymphomas, solid tumors, granulomatous diseases), and radiation-induced underproduction thrombocytopenias. In most of these conditions there is the trilineage suppression of blood counts associated with either decreased numbers of normal-size platelets on blood smear or myelophthisic blood smear abnormalities. There are also distinct pathologic bone marrow changes that always include decreased megakaryocytes.

Hypersplenism can also lead to trilineage decreases in blood cells. In contrast to underproduction thrombocytopenias, however, hypersplenism demonstrates laboratory findings that reflect brisk thrombocytopoiesis, with large platelets on blood smear and increased megakaryocytes in the bone marrow. In addition, 80% of all patients with hypersplenism will have either bedside or radiographic evidence of splenomegaly.

The mainstay of treatments for underproduction thrombocytopenias is transfusing platelets. In addition, there is keen interest in discovering a growth factor that increases endogenous platelet production (analogous to erythropoietin or G-CSF). A recombinant human interleukin, IL-11 ("Neumega"), is one cytokine that has been investigated sufficiently to garner FDA approval. Recombinant human thrombopoietin has been undergoing extensive clinical testing but is not currently available for routine clinical use (12).

IL-11 is indicated for ameliorating chemotherapy-associated thrombocytopenia in patients with solid tumors. It is given at a dose of 50 µg/kg subcutaneously each day starting 24 hours after chemotherapy and ending when the platelet count recovers to a reasonable level (10 to 21 days). Using this program, one should expect to see a modest decrease in the time to platelet recovery (e.g., 9.3 days to reach 50,000/µL versus 13 days for placebo [13]) and a decrease in the percentage of patients who never need a platelet transfusion (70% versus 40% for placebo [13]). There are no data to support its use in leukemia or transplant patients.

Platelet Transfusions

Platelet transfusions are indicated for patients with underproduction thrombocytopenia whenever the platelet count is 30,000/µL or below and there is overt bleeding. Prophylactic platelet transfusion should also be given to patients with counts below 20,000/µL accompanied by wet purpura; patients with counts between 10,000 and 20,000/µL who have petechiae or intractable fevers; and anyone with a platelet count less than 10,000/µL (14,15). Platelet transfusions are also indicated in some situations of thrombocytopenia due to destruction and sequestration. The exceptions to this are TTP, HUS (see Chapter 12), and post-transfusion purpura; in these diseases, platelet transfusions are relatively contraindicated.

There are three types of platelet transfusions: random donor platelets (prepared from whole blood), single donor platelets (prepared by pheresis of a single donor), and HLA-matched platelets (a single donor who is HLA compatible with the recipient). Platelets can be treated with gamma irradiation (which kills lymphocytes and prevents transfusion-associated graft-versus-host disease), ultraviolet B irradiation (which inhibits the presentation of donor antigens and thereby minimizes alloimmunization), and leukoreduction (which minimizes alloimmunization by removing most contaminating leukocytes).

In an unsensitized person, each unit of transfused platelets should result in a post-transfusion increase of blood platelet counts by 5000–10,000/µL. For example, a baseline platelet count of 10,000/µL should increase to somewhere between 50,000/µL and 90,000/µL when 8 units of random donor platelets are administered. When a patient's post-transfusion count fails to achieve such levels, it means that there is alloimmunization, an antiplatelet autoantibody, hypersplenism, or a consumptive process (like DIC or TTP). Fever will also limit the effect of platelet transfusions, so it is best to cool febrile patients before giving them platelets.

Random donor platelets are preferred in almost all settings in which platelet transfusions are used. They should be gamma irradiated whenever they are being given to someone with severe immunosuppression, with a hematological malignancy, or who has received a hematopoietic stem cell transplant procedure. To minimize febrile transfusion reactions, platelets are usually leukoreduced by infusing them through a filter placed at the time of transfusion. Leukoreduction is not optional, however, when platelets are being given to a leukemic patient in whom alloimmunization is expected: these patients, who will need platelets frequently off and on over the course of the next few months while the leukemia is being treated, *must receive either leukofiltered or UV-B-treated platelet transfusions* (16). This decreases the percentage of patients who become refractory to platelet transfusions from 13% down to 3% to 4% (16).

Single-donor platelets are sometimes used to treat patients with alloimmunization, in hopes that a single donor may have platelets that are less alloreactive with the recipient's sensitized lymphocytes. If a good donor is found, it is socially acceptable to solicit weekly (or more frequent) donations. The early use of single-donor platelets does not appear to decrease the frequency of alloimmunization, and it is much more expensive (14).

The use of HLA-matched platelets is reserved for the severely alloimmunized. The match is usually achieved by getting platelets from family members. *Family members generally, and **any potential marrow or peripheral stem cell donor specifically**, cannot direct donations toward their sick family member or provide HLA-matched platelets.* This must be avoided because it will increase the chance of graft rejection and severe graft-versus-host disease.

The best treatment for alloimmunized patients with severe intractable thrombocytopenia and bleeding has not been established. One can administer IVIG before platelets are transfused, hunt for a single donor whose platelets survive in the recipient reasonably well, HLA type the recipient and obtain HLA-compatible platelets, or infuse large quantities of random donor platelets. The latter intervention is the one most often employed to treat dangerous bleeding. When platelet transfusions do not work and the patient is exsanguinating, it is reasonable to administer the antifibrinolytic agent ε-aminocaproic acid at a dose of 24 to 30 grams per day. If you do this, please remember that it can cause acute ureteral obstruction in patients with upper tract urinary bleeding.

Annotated Bibliography

1. Harker LA, Slichter SJ. The bleeding time as a screening test for evaluation of platelet function. N Engl J Med 1972;287:155–159.

   A classic paper that establishes the relationship between bleeding time and platelet count in different diseases.

2. Kaushansky K. Thrombopoietin: the primary regulator of platelet production. Blood 1995;86:419–431.

   A thorough review of the story of thrombopoietin that remains up-to-date save for one detail: investigations of the therapeutic use of TPO have so far been disappointing.

3. The American Society of Hematology ITP Practice Guideline Panel. Diagnosis and treatment of idiopathic thrombocytopenic purpura: recommendations of the American Society of Hematology. Ann Intern Med 1997;126:319–326.

   A concise and useful approach to diagnosing and treating ITP.

4. Oksenhendler E, Bierling P, Chevret S, et al. Splenectomy is safe and effective in human immunodeficiency virus–related immune thrombocytopenia. Blood 1993;82:29–32.

   Splenectomy resulted in ITP remission in 56/68 patients (82%), without any unfavorable effect on the natural history of AIDS. *HIV-associated ITP should be treated identically to idiopathic ITP.*

5. Boumpas DT, Barez S, Klippel JH, Balow JE. Intermittent cyclophosphamide for the treatment of autoimmune thrombocytopenia in systemic lupus erythematosus. Ann Intern Med 1990;112:674–677.

   Cyclophosphamide (0.75–$1.0\,g/m^2$ every 4 weeks) was given with standard dose prednisone to seven patients with systemic lupus erythematosus–associated ITP. All patients responded, and four patients for whom cyclophosphamide was discontinued after 5 or 6 cycles had sustained remissions permitting large reductions in the steroid maintenance dose.

6. Figueroa M, Gehlsen J, Hammond D, et al. Combination chemotherapy in refractory ITP. N Engl J Med 1993;328:1226–1229.

   Ten patients with extremely refractory ITP after splenectomy received several different combinations administered for varying numbers of cycles. There were six complete responses and four of the responders had a durable remission.

7. Calverley DC, Jones GW, Kelton JG. Splenic radiation for corticosteroid-resistant immune thrombocytopenia. Ann Intern Med 1992;116:977–981.

   In this descriptive study, 8 of 11 patients with idiopathic ITP and 1 of 8 patients with secondary ITP had a favorable response to splenic irradiation that lasted at least half a year. The radiation programs were varied, but none used more than 1370 cGy total dose. The most common program was 600 cGy in six doses over 3 weeks, and no patients suffered any radiation toxicity. Despite the results presented, this specific intervention is used very infrequently and should be considered only when surgical splenectomy is contraindicated.

8. McMillan R. Therapy for adults with refractory chronic immune thrombocytopenic purpura. Ann Intern Med 1997;126:307–314.

The best single reference on the subject of clinical aspects of chronic ITP that is currently available.

9. Burrows RF, JG Kelton. Fetal thrombocytopenia and its relation to maternal thrombocytopenia. New Engl J Med 1993;329:1463–1466.

Platelet counts were determined in over 15,000 mothers and their newborn infants. Nineteen infants had counts below 50,000/µL. Of the 19 thrombocytopenic newborns, one was born to one of the 756 mothers with incidental thrombocytopenia; five were born to mothers in the group of 1414 with pregnancy-related hypertension (four with and one without thrombocytopenia); four were born to mothers in the group of 46 with ITP; and nine were born to mothers at risk for alloimmune thrombocytopenia. Of these latter nine infants, six had platelet counts below 20,000/µL, and two out of these six suffered intracranial hemorrhages. There was one stillbirth among the 18 born to the group of 15,471 mothers (0.01% of all women) at risk for alloimmune thrombocytopenia.

10. George JN, Raskob GE, Shah SR, et al. Drug-induced thrombocytopenia; a systematic review of published case reports. Ann Intern Med 1998;129:886–890.

A thorough, up-to-date list of drugs associated with thrombocytopenia. Each is assigned a score of the strength of the evidence of an association.

11. Warkentin TE, Kelton JC. Temporal aspects of heparin-induced thrombocytopenia. N Engl J Med 2001;344:1286–1292.

243 patients with serological evidence of heparin-induced thrombocytopenia were examined. 170 patients developed thrombocytopenia four to ten days after heparin. 73 patients developed thrombocytopenia rapidly (median of 10.5 hours); all had received heparin within the previous 100 days. 7 patients with HIT whose antibody against heparin/platelet factor 4 was lost were subsequently challenged with a brief course of heparin (as therapy for cardiopulmonary or vascular surgery). Serological and clinical HIT did *not* develop in these persons. Most heparin-dependent antibodies vanished 3 months after the discontinuation of heparin.

12. Fanucchi M, Glaspy J, Crawford J, et al. Effects of polyethylene glycol–conjugated recombinant human megakaryocyte growth and development factor (MDGF) on platelet counts after chemotherapy for lung cancer. N Engl J Med 1997;336:404–409.

MDGF (thrombopoietin) was given in a blinded randomized study of 53 patients with lung cancer who were receiving myelosuppressive chemotherapy (carboplatin and paclitaxel). MDGF increased the median nadir platelet count (188,000/µL versus 111,000/µL) and decreased the time for platelet recovery (14 days versus 21 days). The only side effects were nausea, vomiting, and perhaps venous thrombosis.

13. Isaacs C, Robert NJ, Bailey FA, et al. Randomized placebo-controlled study of recombinant human interleukin-11 to prevent chemotherapy-induced thrombocytopenia in patients with breast cancer receiving dose-intensive cyclophosphamide and doxorubicin. J Clin Oncol 1997;15:3368–3377.

Recombinant IL-11 was given to 40 patients after they received high-dose chemotherapy. It decreased the time to platelet count recovery and the need for platelet transfusions. Side effects were edema (63%), dyspnea (50%), conjunctival injection (25%), and pleural effusion (18%).

14. Kruskall M. The perils of platelet transfusion. N Engl J Med 1997;337:1914–1915.

An editorial accompanying two important papers in the same issue of the journal. It concisely summarizes the state of the art and practical clinical standards. If you can read only one thing about platelet transfusion therapy, read this.

15. Rebulla P, Finazzi G, Marangoni F, et al. The threshold for prophylactic platelet transfusions in adults with acute myeloid leukemia. Gruppo Italiano Malattie Ematologiche Maligne dell'Adulto. N Engl J Med 1997;337:1870–1875.

In this study, 255 patients with acute myeloid leukemia were randomized to three different prophylactic transfusion programs: <20,000/μL; 10,000–20,000/μL if temperature was above 38°C in a bleeding patient or an invasive procedure was needed; or <10,000/μL. The risk of major bleeding was the same in all three groups (about 20%). A single fatal intracranial hemorrhage occurred in the <10,000/μL treatment group. Lowering the threshold for prophylactic platelet transfusion to below 10,000/μL reduced the use of platelets by 21.5%.

16. The Trial to Reduce Alloimmunization to Platelets Study Group. Leukocyte reduction and ultraviolet B irradiation of platelets to prevent alloimmunization and refractoriness to platelet transfusions. N Engl J Med 1997;337:1861–1869.

This study randomized 530 patients receiving induction chemotherapy for acute myeloid leukemia to four treatment programs: random-donor platelets, random-donor platelets leukocyte-filtered before transfusion, apheresis single-donor platelets filtered before transfusion, and random-donor platelets treated with UV-B. In all groups the average number of platelet transfusions was about 15, the median exposure to the number of donors was over 50 in all random-donor platelet recipients and 11 in the apheresis group, and refractoriness plateaued about 3 weeks after the transfusion program began. Refractoriness developed in 13% of the random-donor platelet recipients, 3% of the random-donor filtered-platelet recipients, 4% of the single-donor filtered-platelet recipients, and 5% of the recipients of random donor platelets treated with UV-B.

15

Qualitative Platelet Disorders

When a patient has a true hemorrhagic disorder manifested by superficial bleeding, but the workup does not show thrombocytopenia (Chapter 14) or von Willebrand disease (Chapter 16), a qualitative platelet disorder may be possible. A family history suggests a rare inherited syndrome (Table 15.1). When there is no family history, an underlying disease may be affecting platelet function (Table 15.2). Another possibility is *vascular purpura* (Table 15.3). If you still come up empty handed, don't despair! Most qualitative platelet disorders are caused by vague pathophysiologic processes that may never be defined precisely. This does not mean, however, that clinically important diseases will go undiagnosed and untreated. In fact, the diagnosis of a clinically relevant qualitative platelet disorder is simple and the treatment options are straightforward and effective, even if the underlying process remains unknown.

Laboratory Testing

In a patient with a good history of superficial bleeding, the **bleeding time** is the best diagnostic study to objectify that a platelet and/or vessel wall disorder is present. However, the reliability of the bleeding time is notoriously operator-dependent, so it should never be done casually by an inexperienced person. Its reproducibility is the best measure of its accuracy, so it is very important to repeat it whenever it appears spurious or inconsistent with the clinical story. When a patient has a bleeding history and all coagulation studies are normal except the bleeding time (the "isolated elevated bleeding time") it is time to think of a qualitative platelet disorder.

Platelet aggregometry is the next step in the laboratory evaluation used to establish a qualitative platelet disorder. Platelet aggregation testing is usually done on platelet-rich plasma (PRP), isolated from whole blood by centrifugation. For this test, 0.5 mL of PRP is placed in a small siliconized tube warmed to body temperature and containing a small magnetized stir bar. The tube is placed in a chamber that has a light source on one side and a photomultiplier tube on the other side. Platelet aggregation is normalized to light transmission

Table 15.1   Inherited qualitative platelet disorders

Surface receptors
Bernard-Soulier syndrome (GpIb/IX/V deficiency)
Glanzmann's thrombasthenia (GpIIb-IIIa deficiency)
Collagen receptor deficiency
Pseudo (platelet-type) von Willebrand disease

Structural proteins
Wiskott-Aldrich syndrome

Storage organelles
Gray platelet syndrome (α granule deficiency)
Hermansky-Pudlak syndrome (δ granule deficiency)
Chediak-Higashi syndrome (δ granule deficiency)
Thrombocytopenia with absent radii syndrome (δ granule deficiency)
Wiskott-Aldrich syndrome (δ granule deficiency)
$\alpha\delta$ granule deficiency

Signal transduction apparatus
G protein deficiency
Phospholipase C deficiency
Cyclooxygenase deficiency
Thromboxane synthase deficiency

Procoagulant activity
Scott syndrome

Table 15.2   Acquired qualitative platelet disorders

Uremia
Cirrhosis
Myeloproliferative disorders
Myeloma and related disorders
Cardiopulmonary bypass
Drugs
Ethanol

Table 15.3   Causes of vascular purpura

Congenital
Ehlers-Danlos syndrome
Hereditary hemorrhagic telangiectasia

Vasculitis
Henoch-Schönlein purpura
Leukocytoclastic vasculitis
Allergic vasculitis
Serum sickness

Bacteremia
Neisseria sp
Rickettsial diseases
Viral exanthems

Vascular wall fragility
Steroids
Scurvy
Senile purpura
Dysproteinemias

Embolic
Endocarditis
Cholesterol

Mechanical
Puerperal purpura
Factitious purpura

of PRP (0% aggregation) and platelet poor plasma (100% aggregation). Aggregation is started by the addition of a platelet agonist to the aggregation tube, and aggregation is measured in real time by increasing light transmission (or decreasing turbidity—"nephelometry").

Figure 15.1 shows that several physiological agents stimulate normal platelet aggregation. Thrombin, epinephrine, adenosine diphosphate (ADP), and collagen bind to specific receptors that switch platelets "on." Both clopidogrel and ticlopidine interfere with ADP binding to its stimulatory receptor, but only after the liver metabolizes them, so they would not affect platelet aggregation if they were added to the PRP before ADP aggregation was started. On the other hand, partial inhibition of ADP-induced aggregation of PRP from a patient taking one of these drugs is expected. Arachidonic acid is converted to thromboxane A_2 that binds to a receptor and activates platelets. Aspirin blocks this conversion and completely inhibits platelet aggregation in response to arachidonic acid, while often only mildly inhibiting aggregation in response to ADP and epinephrine (see Fig. 15.1E). Ristocetin causes platelets to aggregate by inducing their binding to von Willebrand factor (through the membrane glycoprotein

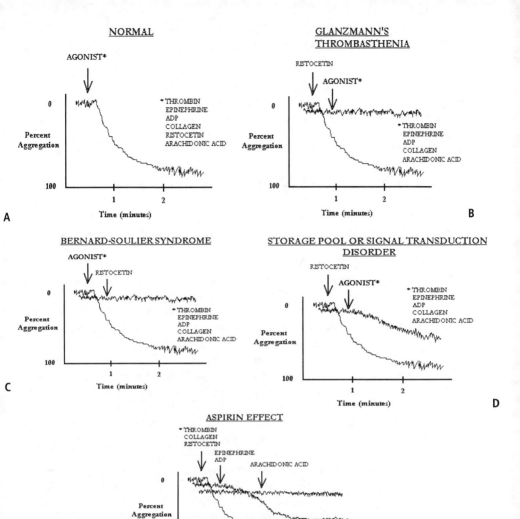

Figure 15.1. Schematic aggregation tracings in qualitative platelet disorders represented by increased light transmission of platelet-rich plasma. Patients with Glanzmann's thrombasthenia, Bernard-Soulier syndrome, storage pool deficiency, or a signal-transduction defect may present with superficial bleeding and an isolated elevated bleeding time. Platelets deficient in the glycoprotein (Gp) IIb-IIIa (integrin αIIbβ3) fail to aggregate in response to all stimuli except ristocetin because normal platelet aggregation in response to all other stimuli depends on fibrinogen binding to GpIIb-IIIa. In contrast, patients with Bernard-Soulier syndrome (BSS) show abnormal aggregation *only* in response to ristocetin, because ristocetin induces von Willebrand factor to bind to platelet GpIb and BSS is due to GpIb deficiency. Storage pool deficiencies and defects in cell activation (or *signal transduction*) show variable changes in aggregation in response to all stimuli except ristocetin. Aspirin sometimes causes mild superficial bleeding with a normal or slightly elevated bleeding time. ASA usually causes decreased platelet aggregation in response to the weak agonists epinephrine and adenosine diphosphate (ADP) and a complete inhibition of arachidonic acid–induced aggregation.

[Gp]Ib complex), and ristocetin-induced aggregation is preserved except when there is a deficiency of GpIb (Bernard-Soulier syndrome) or von Willebrand factor (von Willebrand disease; see Chapter 16). Please note that reliable platelet aggregations require platelet counts to be close to normal, and that aggregation measurements (like bleeding times) done in thrombocytopenic patients are not usually informative.

When platelet aggregometry indicates a functional platelet disorder, determining whether there is a structural basis for it requires two special tools. **Flow cytometry** is used to examine for the presence of surface receptors like GpIb or GpIIb-IIIa. **Electron microscopy** can establish if there are normal α and δ (dense) granules, as well as identify other structural changes like a defective membrane skeleton as found in Wiskott-Aldrich syndrome.

If the functional disorder is not caused by decreased surface receptors or an obvious structural abnormality, or if platelet aggregometry is fairly normal but you are convinced that there is a real qualitative platelet disorder causing bleeding and an isolated elevated bleeding time, there are additional studies usually available in clinical laboratories. Flow cytometry can be used to identify Scott syndrome platelets that lack procoagulant activity (they don't "flip" phosphatidylserine from the inner to outer plasma membrane following activation, and thus binding to *annexin V* is lost after agonist stimulation). Flow cytometry is also used to identify subtler platelet functional disorders that may not cause abnormal aggregation. It can measure platelet activation in whole blood following agonist stimulation. Activation measured by the surface expression of P selectin (CD62P) is a more sensitive test than aggregation, and it may uncover an inherited signal transduction defect or an acquired qualitative abnormality that was not obvious following aggregation measurements. Measuring platelet activation by flow cytometry will also lead to increased false-positive results, so good normal controls are absolutely needed.

Inherited Disorders

The inherited qualitative disorders that cause clinical bleeding and an elevated bleeding time are listed in Table 15.1. Their diagnosis is based on a personal history of bleeding, a family history of bleeding suggesting autosomal recessive transmission, physical examination, and specialized studies. In any patient whose history suggests an inherited qualitative disorder, your first step is to *look for von Willebrand disease*. Why? Because *inherited qualitative bleeding disorders are extremely uncommon and von Willebrand's disease is extremely common*. There are fewer than 100 cases described worldwide for most of the conditions listed in Table 15.1.

Deficiencies of the surface receptors are extremely uncommon. A deficient GpIb complex causes *Bernard-Soulier syndrome* (1). This leads to thrombocytopenia, giant platelets, and absent ristocetin-induced aggregation. *Glanzmann's thrombasthenia* (2) is caused by deficient GpIIb-IIIa, which is the receptor that mediates fibrinogen-dependent platelet aggregation in the aggregometer. Deficiencies of collagen receptors have also been reported in sporadic kindreds.

Pseudo von Willebrand disease is a rare disease caused by mutations in the von Willebrand factor (vWF) binding domain of GpIb that increase its binding to vWF. This leads to enhanced ristocetin-induced aggregation measured by demonstrating aggregation of PRP in response to a low concentration of ristocetin (0.5 mg/mL versus 1.5 mg/mL normally used in aggregation testing).

Many structural proteins are involved in platelet secretion and aggregation. Actin polymerization is absolutely essential. *Wiskott-Aldrich syndrome* (WAS) is an X-linked disease of deficient WAS protein, which regulates actin polymerization. Affected persons have severe thrombocytopenia, immune deficiency, and eczematous dermatitis. Similarly, many signaling proteins (including those that target actin polymerization) are involved in platelet aggregation, and some exceedingly rare disorders that appear to be familial have been described (3). Neither structural abnormalities nor signaling protein disorders are easily diagnosed. They are suspected when there is an isolated unexplained bleeding time with or without abnormal aggregation. The laboratory evaluation requires great specialization (3).

Storage organelle disorders are more easily diagnosed. The abnormality is suspected in patients with isolated unexplained bleeding times who show decreased aggregation in response to more than one agonist (see Fig. 15.1D), although platelet aggregation may be perfectly normal (4). Platelets deficient in α granules (*gray platelet syndrome*) are large and pale, and often decreased in number. Electron microscopy is diagnostic. Platelets deficient in δ (dense) granules can be pinpointed by showing decreased secretion of ATP or radiolabeled serotonin, both of which are stored in δ granules (see Chapter 2). The diagnosis is confirmed by electron microscopy. The *Hermansky-Pudlak syndrome* also causes oculocutaneous albinism, whereas the *thrombocytopenia with absent radii syndrome* affects platelet number and bone (radii) development.

Acquired Disorders

Uremia

Patients with renal failure receiving hemodialysis have a clinical bleeding disorder that can in some cases be severe (5). A qualitative platelet dysfunction disorder is presumed to exist, but testing usually identifies an isolated unexplained bleeding time with no predictable aggregation abnormality. If other coagulation studies are abnormal, patients may be suffering from something in addition to "sick" platelets. There are many hypotheses about the mechanism of uremic platelet dysfunction (5). The most parsimonious and clinically relevant is the *rheology hypothesis*. This proposes that platelet-mediated hemostasis (and its surrogate bleeding time) is affected by the anemia of renal failure: when the red count is low there are fewer platelets pushed to the periphery of blood flow resulting in fewer platelet–vessel wall collisions required for the initiation of platelet plug formation (blood flow is layered like an old-fashioned telescope, with red cells in the center of flow and platelets at the outer layer of flow). In support of this hypothesis is the observation that most patients with uremia whose hematocrit (HCT) is raised toward normal by erythropoietin demonstrate both normalization of the bleeding time and improvement (or resolution) of the bleeding diathesis. If bleeding persists despite an HCT > 36%, platelet transfusions or a nonspecific hemostatic drug such as desmopressin is indicated.

Liver Diseases

Chronic liver diseases, and particularly cirrhosis, cause several problems affecting hemostasis (see Chapter 19). Among these abnormalities is a qualitative platelet abnormality of unknown mechanism and questionable clinical significance (6). The qualitative platelet disorder of liver disease is usually a diagnosis of exclusion. Liver disease often causes thrombocytopenia from sequestration, so the bleeding time may not be helpful. If a patient with cirrhosis is bleeding and the PT, aPTT, thrombin time, and platelet counts are all normal but the bleeding time is elevated, treatment with platelet transfusions or a hemostatic drug is a reasonable consideration.

Myeloproliferative Disorders

The myeloproliferative disorders are chronic myelogenous leukemia, polycythemia vera, myelofibrosis, and essential thrombocytosis. Besides the quantitative stem cell abnormality (overproduction), the diseased stem cells mature abnormally and release platelets that do not work properly. This may result in increased risk for bleeding, as is the usual case for polycythemia vera. Or it may result in an increased risk for arterial (essential thrombocytosis) or venous (polycythemia vera) thrombosis.

In a patient with any one of the myeloproliferative disorders, a clinically significant bleeding disorder is established entirely through observation. The only potential for preemptive strike is in polycythemia vera where, because of the reportedly more predictable a priori bleeding risk, most practitioners avoid aspirin. It should not be avoided, however, if it is indicated for the treatment of arterial thrombosis. Any patient with a myeloproliferative disorder can receive aspirin as long as regular clinical assessments to determine its therapeutic index are maintained.

Myeloma and Related Diseases

High immunoglobulin concentrations in the blood affect platelet function nonspecifically by absorbing onto their surface and interfering with platelet–platelet cohesion. This may be one mechanism by which cirrhotics with panhypergammaglobulinemia acquire a platelet dysfunction syndrome. It also is the likely mechanism by which persons with high levels of monoclonal IgG, IgM, and IgA acquire a qualitative platelet abnormality. This results in an elevated bleeding time and blunted platelet aggregation in response to any or all stimuli. Fortunately, there is no clear relationship between laboratory testing and impaired hemostasis leading to clinically significant bleeding in these diseases. In fact, several types of coagulation disturbances are seen in patients with myeloma (see Chapter 19).

Treatment is generally targeted at minimizing the tumor burden, a process that can cause thrombocytopenia requiring platelet transfusion support. If a patient has severe superficial bleeding associated with impaired platelet responses in vitro, plasmapheresis is sometimes helpful. Platelet transfusions work only if given in sufficient doses to overwhelm the quantity of blood immunoglobulin that will immediately adsorb onto them.

Cardiopulmonary Bypass

Cardiopulmonary bypass (CPB) surgery *always* causes thrombocytopenia within 5 minutes of putting the patient on extracorporeal circulation. The platelet count usually falls by 50% or greater, and it may not rise for several days; usually, it does not fall below 100,000/μL. Yet the bleeding time is usually increased several-fold during CPB and returns to normal within a few hours of coming off CPB. What accounts for this? The cause of the qualitative platelet abnormality acquired during CPB is obscure. It may result in part from platelets getting activated while passing through the pump. This causes "spent" (partially degranulated) platelets to circulate. Clinically significant bleeding in this setting is almost always treated with platelet transfusions.

Drugs, Alcohol, and Foods

A remarkable and fascinating list of medications, drugs, and foods has been associated with platelet dysfunction (7). As with drug-induced ITP, the association suggests causation only when specific criteria are established: there is some sort of temporal relationship between agent and problem, the problem goes away after the agent is stopped, and rechallenge causes recurrence. Unlike ITP, objectifying the problem is more difficult. Ideally, there should be a reproducible increase of the bleeding time and some measurable aggregation abnormality. Because of the notorious inaccuracy of these tests when they are used to go fishing for a problem, one should pursue diagnostic testing only when there is a clear-cut, superficial bleeding disorder and all other causes have been excluded.

There are only a few drugs that are reasonable bets for causing an acquired qualitative platelet abnormality: β-lactam antibiotics (penicillins > cephalosporins), tricyclic antidepressants, phenothiazines, and valproic acid. Aspirin always prolongs the bleeding time, but the prolongation rarely exceeds the upper limit of normal. Aspirin causes bleeding only in persons with an underlying defect of hemostasis such as von Willebrand disease. Alcohol, which can poison many hemostatic reactions, will prolong the bleeding time and inhibit platelet aggregation. Whether this affects hemostasis in vivo is unknown (but is doubtful). It actually may have a salutary effect on arterial thrombosis, and this is one mechanism suggested for the cardiovascular benefits observed with modest daily ethanol intake.

Management

Bleeding associated with a qualitative platelet disorder is usually managed by giving platelet transfusions. Dosing aims to raise the baseline count by about 30,000–60,000/μL (about 6 units of random-donor platelets; see Chapter 14). In some cases transfused platelets acquire the functional abnormality immediately (e.g., when there are high levels of immunoglobulin) and in some cases the acquired abnormality gradually affects transfused platelets (e.g., when carbenicillin is continued). The obvious measure employed to prevent the acquisition of a functional platelet defect in transfused platelets is, whenever possible, to eliminate the suspected culprit.

There are also non-transfusional modalities for treating patients with qualitative platelet diseases (8). The two that have been investigated carefully in uremia are desmopressin (DDAVP) and conjugated estrogens. Many practitioners extrapolate from these studies that these agents are also useful for patients with other qualitative platelet disorders. Such an extrapolation can be justified as long as one understands how these agents work, and what their side effects and therapeutic limitations are. Most importantly, those who use desmopressin and/or estrogen to treat an isolated unexplained bleeding time must recognize that there are no data to support or refute their use for this indication, so the therapeutic target must be the prevention or cessation of clinical bleeding. The bleeding time should only be used as a therapeutic target when it is an established surrogate for clinical bleeding risk.

Desmopressin is an analogue of vasopressin. Desmopressin binds to specific endothelial cell receptors and stimulates their release of large vWF multimers. Most vascular endothelium synthesizes vWF. Some vWF is constitutively released adluminally into the blood and abluminally into the vessel wall. The remaining vWF is stored in granules designated *Weibel-Palade bodies*. When desmopressin is administered, stored vWF is released. The released vWF is relatively enriched in the larger, most hemostatically effective multimers. vWF multimers function as a kind of local "glue" that nonspecifically enhances hemostasis by enhancing the initial interaction between platelets and the damaged vessel wall. Plasma vWF concentrations can triple within 60 minutes of desmopressin administration, and elevated bleeding times normalize within 4 to 6 hours in about 75% of uremic patients given standard doses. Dosing is usually at 12- to 24-hour intervals, and the therapeutic response disappears after three to five doses due to exhaustion of stored vWF. Stores are replenished within 5 to 7 days after stopping the desmopressin.

Desmopressin is administered intravenously, subcutaneously, or intranasally (Table 15.4). Its principal side effect is water retention, so it must be used with caution in patients with heart failure or liver disease with ascites. It may also cause vasospasm and can theoretically trigger platelet thrombosis in diseased

Table 15.4   Hemostatic drugs

DRUG	INDICATION	DOSE	ONSET	DURATION
Desmopressin	Acute bleeding	0.3 μg/kg (intravenous, subcutaneous)	30–60 minutes	6–12 hours
	Before biopsy or emergency surgery	300 μg (intranasal) every 12–24 hours for 4 to 5 doses	60–90 minutes	6–12 hours
Conjugated Estrogens	Chronic, recurrent bleeding	0.6 mg/kg infusion every day for 5 to 7 days	7 days	2 weeks
	Before elective surgery	50 mg orally every day for 5 to 7 days		

arteries, so it should be used judiciously in patients who have active coronary artery disease, and should probably be avoided in cases of unstable angina and myocardial infarction. Desmopressin is used routinely to elevate vWF levels when patients with von Willebrand disease require it (see Chapter 16); because vWF is a carrier protein for factor VIII, desmopressin is also used to treat mild hemophilia A (see Chapter 17).

Conjugated estrogens also nonspecifically enhance hemostasis. Their mechanism of action may also involve vWF. They increase vWF levels by increasing the constitutive synthesis and release of vWF. This mechanism predicts that conjugated estrogens have a longer lag in onset and a longer therapeutic phase. Such predictions have been validated by observing that uremic patients treated with standard-dose conjugated estrogens (see Table 15.4) have their elevated bleeding time reduced after about 1 week, and that the reduction lasts an additional 2 weeks. Conjugated estrogens used to treat a qualitative platelet disorder are given only as a pulse of five to seven daily doses, and with this schedule no side effects have been observed.

Annotated Bibliography

1. Lopez JA, Andrews RK, Afshar-Kharghan V, Berndt MC. Bernard Soulier syndrome. Blood 1998;91:4397–4418.

   A thorough review of the clinical manifestations, biology, and genetics of inherited deficiencies of the platelet glycoprotein Ib/IX/V complex.

2. Nurden AT. Inherited abnormalities of platelets. Thromb Haemost 1999;82:468–480.

   A review of several inherited qualitative platelet disorders, emphasizing pathophysiology and Glanzmann's thrombasthenia. It subcategorizes the abnormalities into a clinically identifiable group designated *giant platelet syndromes*. These include *Bernard-Soulier syndrome*, the *May-Hegglin anomaly* (with thrombocytopenia and granulocyte Dohle bodies), *Mediterranean familial macrothrombocytopenia*, *Montreal platelet syndrome*, and *Epstein's syndrome*.

3. Rao AK, Gabbeta J. Congenital disorders of platelet signal transduction. Arterioscler Thromb Vasc Biol 2000;20:285–289.

A detailed review of the subject, with interesting speculation that the majority of persons with superficial bleeding and an isolated unexplained bleeding time will turn out to have a platelet-signaling defect. Time will tell.

4. Nieuwenhuis HK, Akkerman J-WN, Sixma JJ. Patients with a prolonged bleeding time and normal aggregation tests may have storage pool deficiency: studies on 106 patients. Blood 1987;70:620–623.

This is an excellent study of 106 patients with objectively established δ storage pool deficiency. Of this group, 22% had normal platelet aggregation.

5. Weigert AL, Schafer AI. Uremic bleeding: pathogenesis and therapy. Am J Med Sci 1998;316:94–104.

A review of uremic bleeding, including clinical manifestations unique to dialysis patients and specific guidelines for treatment based on our understanding of the pathophysiology of the acquired qualitative platelet abnormalities in uremia.

6. Ballard HS, Marcus AJ. Platelet aggregation in portal cirrhosis. Arch Intern Med 1976;136:316–319.

This review of the state of the subject was written in 1976, and nothing more, or more interesting, has been produced over the ensuing quarter of a century. It describes three factors contributing to platelet dysfunction in liver disease: 1) fibrin degradation products that interfere with fibrinogen cross-linking platelets (definite small role), 2) abnormal fibrinogen that does not bridge GpIIb-IIIa very well (possible small role), and 3) something else (definite large role).

7. George JN, Shattil SJ. The clinical importance of acquired abnormalities of platelet function. New Engl J Med 1991;324:27–42.

In this exhaustive review of medications, drugs, foods, and other things that affect platelet function, there is a wonderful table listing each agent's in vitro versus in vivo effects. If you have a patient with bleeding and an isolated unexplained bleeding time, with or without abnormal aggregation, cross-reference this table with their medication list and a review of systems. And if there is no cross-reference between a patient's history and the actual list, you should use one other fact implicit in this article: *anything goes*. Figure out if stopping an agent reverses the clinical and laboratory abnormalities. And if it does, inform the FDA and write it up.

8. Mannucci PM. Hemostatic drugs. New Engl J Med 1998;339:245–253.
   A useful review of drugs used to improve hemostasis in patients with
   qualitative platelet abnormalities and several other more common clinical
   conditions. The drugs presented are antifibrinolytic agents (ε-aminocaproic
   acid and tranexamic acid), the serine protease inhibitor aprotinin,
   desmopressin, and conjugated estrogens.

16

Von Willebrand Disease

Von Willebrand disease (vWD) should be placed at the top of every list of differential diagnoses for a superficial bleeding disorder, particularly menorrhagia (1). The family history need not be obvious, as disease penetrance of the most common form of vWD (type 1 vWD) is unpredictable (Table 16.1). Variable penetrance of type 1 vWD is especially true among women in their childbearing years because plasma levels of von Willebrand factor (vWF) wax and wane with levels of cycling estrogens throughout the menstrual period. How common is vWD? It is the most common bleeding problem on earth. If one considers that the prevalence of vWD in the United States is at least 1 out of every 1000 people, there are over 200,000 affected persons in this country alone. Although this is far less than the number of persons suffering from diseased coronary arteries, it is large enough to force the emphasis of two points. 1) Every family practitioner or general internist will have a patient with vWD in their practice at some point in time. 2) No one knows what selective advantage the vWD genes provide, but there must be some basis for their persistence during the evolution of *Homo sapiens*.

Biology of von Willebrand Factor

Von Willebrand factor (vWF) may be the most important hemostatic protein. It is synthesized only in vascular endothelium and megakaryocytes. It is constitutively released from the endothelium both adluminally and abluminally so that it circulates in plasma and interdigitates itself as a solid constituent of the vascular subendothelial extracellular matrix. It is also stored in endothelial cell Weibel-Palade bodies and platelet alpha granules, where it is available for rapid release following cell stimulation. It has a versatile primary structure (it has binding domains for collagen, heparin, factor VIII, and platelet glycoproteins Ib and IIb-IIIa) and it multimerizes into disulfide-linked (very strong bond) polymers of up to 100 individual vWF molecules (called *multimers*). These structural attributes result in a protein "monster" that, at any given time, can grab onto literally hundreds of other proteins. And this monster sits guard over our microvasculature, vigilantly attaching itself to exposed subendothelium and

Table 16.1   The classification of von Willebrand disease

TYPE	GENETICS	CLINICAL FEATURES	LABORATORY FEATURES	MECHANISM	TREATMENT
1 (~70%)	Prevalence 1–30/1000; autosomal dominant; 60% penetrance	Mild–moderate bleeding	vWF:Ag, ristocetin cofactor activity and FVIII levels 20–50%; multimers normal	Some missense mutations in vWF gene; some heterozygous type 3.	Desmopressin Conjugated estrogens Humate-P
2A (~10%)	Prevalence 1–3/10,000 Autosomal dominant > recessive; full penetrance	Mild–moderate bleeding	vWF:Ag, ristocetin cofactor activity and FVIII levels variably decreased; no large multimers	1) Defective intracellular transport. 2) Increased plasma proteolysis.	Humate-P *(Desmopressin and conjugated estrogens may not work.)*
2B (~5%)	Prevalence < 1/10,000	Mild–moderate bleeding and mild thrombocytopenia	vWF:Ag, ristocetin cofactor activity and FVIII levels variably decreased; decreased large multimers; ↑ RIPA	Increased binding to Gplb due to missense mutations in vWF gene Gplb binding (A1) domain.	Conjugated estrogens Humate-P *(Desmopressin is contraindicated.)*
2M (very rare)	Prevalence unknown but very low (case reports only); autosomal dominant	Variable bleeding	vWF:Ag and FVIII levels variably decreased; normal multimers; very decreased ristocetin cofactor activity	Decreased vWF binding to Gplb due to missense mutations in vWF gene Gplb binding (A1) domain.	Humate-P
2N (rare)	Prevalence unknown except in specific populations. "Autosomal hemophilia"	Mild–moderate bleeding; hemophilia in homozygotes	vWF:Ag and ristocetin cofactor activity variably decreased; multimers normal; FVIII levels disproportionately low	Missense mutations in vWF's factor VIII binding domain eliminate its factor VIII carrier function.	Humate-P
3 (~5%)	Prevalence 1–5/1,000,000 Autosomal recessive	Severe bleeding	vWF:Ag, ristocetin cofactor activity and FVIII levels almost undetectable	Deletions, point mutations, and missense mutations eliminate vWF transcription or translation.	Humate-P

Abbreviations: RIPA = ristocetin-induced platelet aggregation.

then grabbing onto platelets' GpIb receptors while they shoot past. It then tethers platelets to areas of vessel wall damage, stimulates platelet activation, and forms the physical connection between activated GpIIb-IIIa molecules on adjacent platelets that results in their aggregation (2). This plugs the damaged vessel and initiates the repair process.

The platelet-subendothelial and platelet-platelet connections possess great tensile strength, capable of withstanding the greatly elevated pathological shearing forces generated in constricted coronary arteries (shearing forces that sweep away all fibrin deposition and tear apart any interplatelet fibrinogen bridging). As the platelet thrombus grows and blood flow slows, the soluble coagulation reactions commence generating a fibrin barrier. This phase of hemostasis is enhanced by factor VIII delivered directly to the nascent thrombus by its carrier molecule vWF.

Clinical Aspects of von Willebrand Disease

Superficial bleeding is the hallmark of vWD. Despite vWF being a carrier molecule for factor VIII, a hemophilia-like bleeding disorder is rare and only seen in patients with type 2N and severe (type 3) vWD (see Table 16.1). Epistaxis and menorrhagia that begin at menarche occur in at least two-thirds of all patients with vWD. Bleeding after tooth extraction and easy bruising occur in the majority of vWD cases. Excessive bleeding following minor trauma, gingival bleeding, postoperative bleeding, and bleeding at delivery occur in over 25% of all cases. Joint bleeding is uncommon, occurring in less than 10% of vWD cases overall and only about one-third of type 3 vWD patients (versus 90% of patients with severe hemophilia). Bleeding in vWD patients is often intermittent and can be provoked by aspirin use. The diagnosis of vWD is supported by an elevated bleeding time, but a normal bleeding time in no way excludes the diagnosis of vWD, as it is frequently normal in all except type 3 disease. Similarly, the aPTT is usually normal in all except types 2N and 3 vWD.

vWD Diagnosis and Classification

vWD classification is shown in Table 16.1. The classification is based on laboratory studies that are listed in Table 16.2. The vWF:Ag is the quantity of immunoreactive vWF protein, usually measured by an ELISA. The ristocetin cofactor activity is a functional assay of vWF that measures the capacity of a person's plasma to support ristocetin-induced aggregation of control platelets. Ristocetin induces vWF to bind to platelet GpIb; the vWF binding to adjacent platelets causes aggregation in a conventional platelet aggregometer (see Chapter 15). Ristocetin aggregation measures the capacity of a patient's platelet-rich plasma to aggregate in response to conventional (1.5 mg/mL) and subthreshold (0.5 mg/mL) concentrations of ristocetin. Multimers are analyzed by protein separation in agarose followed by vWF identification by immunoblotting.

Table 16.2 The laboratory diagnosis of von Willebrand disease

TYPE	vWF:Ag LEVEL	FVIII LEVEL	RISTOCETIN COFACTOR ACTIVITY (vWF:RCo)	RISTOCETIN AGGREGATION	MULTIMERS
1	<50%	<50%			
2A	Low (variable)	Low (variable)			
2B	Low (variable)	Low (variable)			
3	~0	~0			

Abbreviations: PPP = platelet-poor plasma; PRP = platelet-rich plasma.

The diagnosis of type 1 vWD is confounded by variability in measuring vWF:Ag and the ristocetin cofactor activity. Variability is affected by the menstrual cycle (estrogen elevates vWF levels), blood type (individuals with type O blood have 15% lower vWF levels), and inflammation (vWF is elevated in disease states that cause endothelial cell damage). As a result of this variability, which is associated with perhaps a 40% false-negative result rate, testing with the standard battery of measurements in Table 16.2 is often repeated several times before the diagnosis of vWD is confirmed or excluded.

Treatment of vWD

The treatment of vWD is straightforward because there is a limited selection of interventions available. Fortunately, the available treatments are simple to implement, and are fairly safe and effective. The treatments available in the United States are desmopressin, purified factor VIII/vWF (Humate-P, Aventis Behring), antifibrinolytics, conjugated estrogens, and fibrin glue.

Desmopressin

Desmopressin is administered intravenously, subcutaneously, or intranasally (see Table 15.4). About 80% of type 1, 25% of type 2A, and no type 3 vWD patients will respond to desmopressin. Desmopressin is contraindicated in type 2B vWD because it causes increased mutant vWF binding to platelets and has precipitated thrombocytopenia, which is believed to be a harbinger of thrombotic risk.

Desmopressin is indicated for bleeding episodes, including menorrhagia, and can be given every 12 to 24 hours for a total of four to six doses before tachyphylaxis develops. Desmopressin is also effective in preventing bleeding associated with surgery and dental procedures. A test dose of desmopressin is usually given before elective surgery or invasive procedures. To establish the drug's efficacy, vWF:Ag and/or a bleeding time are measured 4 to 6 hours after a test dose of desmopressin. When desmopressin works, vWF goes up three-fold to sixfold and the prolonged bleeding time is reduced to normal.

Humate-P

Humate-P is the only factor VIII/vWF preparation that has been approved by the U.S. Food and Drug Administration for replacement therapy in vWF. Humate-P is manufactured from pooled plasma that has been heat treated for 10 hours at 60°C. Other plasma-derived concentrates of factor VIII are also clinically effective agents, but recombinant factor VIII and monoclonal antibody purified FVIII should not be used because they do not contain vWF, and solvent-detergent–treated products cannot be used because large vWF multimers are lost during the treatment process (3). Humate-P is indicated for treating vWD when desmopressin does not work.

The dosage is based on a volume of distribution of about one-half of the plasma compartment, a duration of activity of vWF of at least 24 hours, and the convention that 1 mL of normal plasma contains 1 IU of ristocetin cofactor activity (vWF:RCo). However, the bleeding time correction wanes before the levels of vWF:RCo decrease, which makes the dosing principles more empiric than formulaic. Current recommendations (1) are found in Table 16.3.

Hemostatic Agents

Hemostatic agents are also used routinely to treat patients with vWD. Menorrhagia can be treated with an antifibrinolytic agent like ε-aminocaproic acid given at a dose of 6 grams, orally, four times a day. Menorrhagia may improve dramatically with the use of oral contraceptives. Nonmenstrual, self-limited minor bleeding sometimes improves with conjugated estrogens (see Chapter 15). Dental procedures in desmopressin unresponsive patients can sometimes be managed without factor replacement by using an antifibrinolytic agent plus the application of a fibrin sealant. The only fibrin sealant currently available in the United States is Tiseel (Baxter).

Recombinant Activated Factor VII

Recombinant activated factor VII (FVIIa) is probably the best treatment available for patients with type 3 or acquired vWD (see below) who have severe bleeding, who require major surgery, or who are at parturition, but have circulating anti-vWF antibodies that preclude the use of Humate-P. FVIIa (Novo-Seven, Novo Nordisk) is given as a dose of 90 μg/kg every 3 to 4 hours until bleeding or its risk subsides.

Acquired vWD

The acquired von Willebrand syndrome (AvWS) is a heterogeneous group of diseases that cause a late-onset superficial bleeding disorder in persons who do not have a personal or family history of bleeding (4). Laboratory investigation will yield test results consistent with vWD. The majority of cases develop in patients with myeloma and related disorders. Other causes include myeloproliferative disorders, lymphoproliferative disorders, connective tissue disorders, and hypothyroidism (4). The pathogenesis usually is hazy and attributed to adsorption of vWF (onto tumor cells), defective synthesis (hypothyroidism), or exaggerated proteolysis of vWF (myeloproliferative disorders). Only a small fraction (<15%) of AvWS cases is caused by autoantibodies to vWF.

The best course of therapy is to reverse the primary process causing the AvWS. When this doesn't work, the treatment for AvWS is much the same as for inherited vWD, but the standard interventions used for vWD are not as predictably effective for AvWS. High-dose intravenous immunoglobulin (0.5–1.0 g/kg) may be effective in AvWS associated with plasma cell or B cell lymphoproliferative disorders.

Table 16.3   Treatment recommendations for von Willebrand disease

SITUATION	TREATMENT RECOMMENDATION
Major Surgery/Bleed	
Mild type 1 vWD (vWF:RCo > 30%)	Target is nadir vWF:RCo > 50%. • Load with 40–60 IU/kg Humate-P. • Continue 40–50 IU/kg every 8–12 hours for 3 days, then 40–50 IU/kg per day for 7 days. • Monitor vWF:RCo and FVIII levels Example: vWF level of 0.35 IU/mL (35%); weight of 60 kg. Give 3000 IU Humate-P load, followed by 2400 IU every 12 hours for 3 days, followed by 2400 IU every 24 hours for 3 to 4 days.
Moderate or severe type 1 vWD (vWF:RCo < 30%)	Target is nadir vWF:RCo > 50%. • Load with 50–75 IU/kg Humate-P. • Continue 40–60 IU/kg every 8–12 hours for 3 days, then 40–60 IU/kg per day for 7 days. • Monitor vWF:RCo levels.
Type 2 or 3 vWD	Target is nadir vWF:RCo > 50% and/or FVIII > 0.5 IU/mL. • Load with 50–75 IU/kg Humate-P. • Continue 40–60 IU/kg every 8–12 hours for 3 days, then 40–60 IU/kg per day for 7 days. • Monitor vWF:RCo levels.
Minor Surgery/Bleed	
All types (1, 2, and 3) vWD	Target is vWF:RCo > 30% and/or FVIII > 0.3 IU/mL. • Administer 40–75 IU/kg Humate-P for only one or two doses.
Dental Procedures	
All types (1, 2, and 3) vWD	Target is vWF:RCo > 40% and/or FVIII > 0.4 IU/mL during procedure and for 6 hours afterward. • Administer 40–60 IU/kg Humate-P once. • Administer 0.3 µg/kg desmopressin once or twice.
Delivery	
Types 1 and 2 vWD	• Check level of vWF:RCo and FVIII before parturition *If* vWF:RCo > 50% and/or FVIII > 0.5 IU/mL (50 IU/dL): • No treatment. *If* vWF:RCo is between 20 and 50% and/or FVIII is between 0.2 and 0.5 IU/mL: • Monitor; use desmopressin postpartum only if there is excessive bleeding. *If* vWF:RCo < 20% and/or FVIII < 0.2 IU/mL: Target is >50% activity or >0.5 IU/mL. • Load with 50–75 IU/kg Humate-P. • Continue 40–60 IU/kg every 8–12 hours for 3 days
Type 3 vWD	Target is nadir vWF:RCo > 50%. • Load with 50–75 IU/kg Humate-P. • Continue 40–60 IU/kg every 8–12 hours for 3 days.

Annotated Bibliography

1. Sadler JE, Mannucci PM, Berntop E, et al. Impact, diagnosis and treatment of von Willebrand disease. Thromb Haemost 2000;84:160–174.

   This is the complete, up-to-date primer on von Willebrand disease generated by an august international group of physician scientists.

2. Kroll MH, Hellums JD, McIntire LV, et al. Platelets and shear stress. Blood 1996;85:1525–1541.

   A review of blood flow effects on platelet function and how von Willebrand factor works under rheologic conditions that prevent both fibrin deposition and the formation of fibrinogen bridges between platelets.

3. Mannucci PM, Tenconi PM, Castaman G, Rodeghiero F. Comparison of four virus-inactivated plasma concentrates for treatment of severe von Willebrand disease: a cross-over randomized trial. Blood 1992;79:3130–3137.

   This is an important report that forced the medical community to come up with vWF replacement therapy better than cryoprecipitate. The data in this paper are now (fortunately) anachronistic, cryoprecipitate is no longer routinely used in developed countries, and the U.S. FDA has recently approved a concentrate for use in vWD patients who do not respond to desmopressin.

4. Veyradier A, Jenkins CSP, Fressinaud E, Meyer D. Acquired von Willebrand syndrome: from pathophysiology to management. Thromb Haemost 2000;84:175–182.

   Reviews the clinical experience of these investigators and general information based on their analysis of the literature. The acquired von Willebrand syndrome is very rare; fewer than 500 documented cases have been identified worldwide.

17

Hemophilia and Other Coagulation Factor Deficiencies

Clinical Overview

Most inherited coagulation factor deficiencies lead to bleeding of the joints, muscles, and oral mucosa. Newborns with an unrecognized severe deficiency suffer cephalohematomas, excessive circumcision bleeding, and, rarely, intracranial bleeding. The diagnosis is usually based on screening studies (most commonly an elevated aPTT), mixing studies (the aPTT corrects with mixing), and a clotting assay that measures the capacity of the patient's plasma to normalize the elevated clotting time observed when factor-deficient plasma is used as the substrate (testing that resolves deficiencies of 30% or less). The conventional nomenclature for hemophilia—factor VIII and factor IX deficiency—as well as all coagulation factor deficiency states, defines normal coagulation factor activity as that present in 100 dL of plasma (= 100% or 100 IU/dL or 1 IU/mL). Clinical experience (which refreshes one's appreciation for the elegant fine-tuning of our hemostatic system) establishes that severe hemophilia is less than 1% activity, moderate hemophilia is 2% to 5% activity, and mild hemophilia is 6% to 40%. Similar ranges are applied to other factor deficiencies.

Severe hemophiliacs have extensive spontaneous bleeding, including joint bleeds that lead to crippling arthropathy. Moderately severe hemophiliacs have spontaneous bleeding, occasional hemarthroses, and severe surgical or traumatic bleeding. Mild hemophiliacs with factor levels between 6% and 20% have mild spontaneous bleeding but will suffer excessive bleeding following provocation. Mild hemophiliacs with factor levels greater than 20% may be perfectly normal, only suffering bleeding after major surgery or trauma.

The two major challenges that face a practitioner after the diagnosis of an inherited coagulation factor deficiency is made are 1) optimizing treatment to optimize the quality of life for the patient, and 2) genetic counseling. These issues are interwoven into the descriptions that follow. Please note that among all newborns that inherit hemophilia, including those with severe disease, their expectations should be that they would live out a normal life span. However, their capacity to live a normal life is inextricably linked to the activity of their physicians and the resources provided by the health care system into which they are born (1).

Factor VIII Deficiency (Hemophilia A)

Hemophilia A is caused by mutations of the factor VIII (FVIII) gene on the X-chromosome. Approximately 1 male child out of 5000 is affected by hemophilia A. Over 200 mutations in the large and complex FVIII gene lead to inadequate synthesis of FVIII. Fortunately, about one-half of all hemophilia A is due to an inversion of intron 22, which simplifies the diagnostic and genetic counseling workups. Only after such a mutation has been excluded should the FVIII gene be examined for some other mutation, which can be applied in a pedigree analysis for finding female carriers and making prenatal diagnoses of hemophilia A. Figure 17.1 shows a flow sheet that represents a case description of applying genetics to hemophilia A.

Just as forest fire prevention is the foundation for managing our national parks, bleeding prevention must be considered the primary approach for managing severe hemophiliacs. Standard treatment of bleeding in persons with moderate or severe hemophilia A depends mainly on the target FVIII level established through empirical methods (Table 17.1). Such standard treatment protocols must be put into a broader context of optimal therapy. And because the safety of FVIII replacement therapy can now be taken for granted, the therapeutic index of all available treatments must be considered within the context of medical economics as well as clinical pharmacology: each of the agents listed in Table 17.2 costs between $0.90 and $1.30 per unit wholesale.

The treatment of mild hemophilia usually involves only desmopressin, administered parenterally, subcutaneously, or intranasally (see Table 15.4). The treatment of moderate or severe hemophilia involves administering FVIII.

Newborn boy suffers excessive bleeding post circumcision → Uncertain family history → aPTT elevated → Corrects with normal plasma 1:1 mix → Factor VIII level 3% (3 IU/dl) → Plasma DNA extracted → DNA analyzed by PCR* for intron 22 inversion → (+) → DNA of mother, father and sister tested → Only mother carries intron 22 inversion → Maternal grandmother and aunts are tested → Mother becomes pregnant → chorionic villous sample at 10 weeks reveals unaffected male child → Routine term vaginal delivery

* polymerase chain reaction

Figure 17.1.   A fictitious case study to show how genetic testing for hemophilia A can be applied to prenatal diagnosis. (PCR = polymerase chain reaction.)

Table 17.1   **Standard treatment for moderate and severe hemophilia A**

BLEEDING	TARGET FVIII LEVEL (IU/dL OR % NORMAL)	DOSE INTERVAL	OTHER ISSUES
Early hemarthrosis, muscle bleed, or oral bleed	20–40	12–24 hours	Treat up to 3 days; rest/immobilization/PT.
Extensive hemarthrosis, or muscle or oral bleed	40–60	12–24 hours	Treat up to 3 days; rest/immobilization/PT.
Life-threatening bleed (head, throat, GI, GU)	60–100	8–12 hours	Treat until threat resolves.
Epistaxis	80–100	8–12 hours	Drop target to 30% after bleeding stops; continue until healed.
Tooth extraction	60–80	Once	Use with antifibrinolytic agent begun within 1 hour of procedure (e.g., ε-aminocaproic acid 100 mg/kg) and continued for 3 to 5 days (e.g., 6 grams ε-aminocaproic acid, orally, four times a day).
Minor surgery	60–80	Once	Repeat only if clinical suspicion of postoperative bleed.
Major surgery	100	8–24 hours	Maintain 100% for 1 to 2 days then 30–50% until healing complete.
Brain bleed or surgery	100	8–12 hours	Maintain 100% for 5 days and then 50% for 5 to 10 more days.

Abbreviations: GI = gastrointestinal; GU = genitourinary; PT = physical therapy.

The dose of FVIII is calculated by this equation:

$$(\text{Target FVIII level} - \text{Baseline FVIII level}) \times \frac{\text{Weight in kg}}{2}$$

The denominator 2 is used because the volume of distribution of FVIII is less than plasma volume, probably due to vWF binding and delivery to sites of hemostatic need. The half-life of FVIII, including replacement FVIII, is about 12 hours, so treatment usually involves at least two daily doses. FVIII infusions are also used. Continuous infusion provides the advantage of eliminating trough levels (important for severe bleeding or major surgery) and may actually decrease the total daily dose required to achieve effective hemostasis. The initial infusion rate simply aims to administer the target total daily dose over 24 hours of continuous infusion, with adjustments based on FVIII level measurement.

Table 17.2 Factor VIII products for treatment of hemophilia A

	ALPHANATE	ANTIHEMOPHILIC FACTOR-M	HELIXATE	HEMOFIL M	HUMATE-P	KOATE-DVI	KOATE-HP	KOGENATE	MONOCLATE-P	RECOMBINATE
	Alpha	American Red Cross	Centeon	Baxter	Centeon	Bayer	Bayer	Bayer	Centeon	Baxter
	Solvent-detergent plasma-derived	Solvent-detergent-treated plasma-derived by monoclonal antibody affinity purification	Recombinant + human albumin + trace mouse IgG + trace hamster proteins	Solvent-detergent-treated plasma-derived by monoclonal antibody affinity purification	Heat-treated plasma-derived	Solvent-detergent and heat-treated plasma-derived	Solvent-detergent plasma-derived	Recombinant + human albumin + trace mouse IgG + trace hamster proteins	Heat-treated plasma-derived by monoclonal immunoaffinity purification	Recombinant + bovine albumin + trace mouse IgG + trace hamster proteins
	$T_{1/2}$ = 9–14 hours	$T_{1/2}$ = 14 hours	$T_{1/2}$ = 15 hours	$T_{1/2}$ = 14 hours	$T_{1/2}$ = 12 hours	$T_{1/2}$ = 16 hours	$T_{1/2}$ = 9–14 hours	$T_{1/2}$ = 16 hours	$T_{1/2}$ = 17 hours	$T_{1/2}$ = 14 hours
	vWF multimers absent	No vWF	Monoclonal antibody purification step; no vWF	No vWF	Also used for vWF replacement	Double viral inactivation (DVI), vWF multimers absent	High potency (HP); vWF multimers absent	Monoclonal antibody purification step; no vWF	No vWF	Monoclonal antibody purification step; vWF is co-expressed and stabilizes FVIII
	1 IU/kg raises FVIII level by 2.0%	1 IU/kg raises FVIII level by 2.0%	1 IU/kg raises FVIII level by 2.0%	1 IU/kg raises FVIII level by 2.0%	1 IU/kg raises FVIII level by 2.0%	1 IU/kg raises FVIII level by 2.0%	1 IU/kg raises FVIII level by 2.5%	1 IU/kg raises FVIII level by 2.0%	1 IU/kg raises FVIII level by 2.0%	1 IU/kg raises FVIII level by 2.0%

Abbreviations: IgG = immunoglobulin gamma; $T_{1/2}$ = half-life.

To give an example of a typical case, neurosurgery in a hemophiliac requires a target FVIII level of 100% activity (100 IU/dL) for about 4 days, followed by an additional 10 days at 50% activity level. Replacement for a 60 kg severely deficient person is calculated as

$$(100-0)\times\frac{60}{2} = 3000\,\text{IU (about \$3000.00)}$$

given every 8 to 12 hours the first 96 hours after the operation. Dosing and interval adjustments are made based on FVIII level measurements. If a 14-day course is required, one can anticipate a total of approximately 10 doses of 3000 IU and approximately 10 to 20 doses at 1500 IU for a total cost of at least $50,000.00.

In an attempt to improve the quality of life for patients with severe hemophilia, the World Health Organization and World Federation of Hemophilia have written the following policy:

Since the main goal is to prevent joint bleeding and its sequelae, prophylaxis should be considered optimal management for persons with severe Hemophilia A or B. Treatment should begin at the age of 1–2 years and be continued indefinitely. Where prophylaxis is not feasible or appropriate, on-demand therapy should be given.

The National Hemophilia Foundation of the United States endorses this policy. Prophylaxis seeks to convert severe into moderate hemophiliacs by administering FVIII to maintain levels above 1%. A common program used to accomplish this is 20–40 IU FVIII/kg body weight, three times per week, with dose modification that provides the lowest total annual dose required to maintain FVIII over 1%. This type of program is reasonably effective at decreasing bleeding episodes (it decreases bleeding, including joint bleeds, by about 60%). It also uses much more factor and is more expensive: a mean annual consumption of 3000 IU/kg versus 900 IU/kg for on-demand therapy (2).

Preliminary results suggest that joint symptoms and preservation of joint function are likely to be improved by prophylactic FVIII programs. Various modifications are being investigated, including the continuous infusion of FVIII, but it will be years before the optimal management of children with severe hemophilia is achieved, even in developed countries.

Including children on prophylaxis, 30% of hemophilia A patients who receive human FVIII will develop an inhibitor. The risk appears to be about the same among all of the products listed in Table 17.2. Risk is greatest in persons whose deficiency is due to large deletions in the FVIII gene. When an inhibitor develops, it is quantified in *Bethesda units* (BU); 1 BU is defined as the amount of antibody per milliliter that inactivates 50% of the FVIII activity in a 1:1 mix of normal, pooled plasma with the affected person's plasma. A *low responder* is someone with an inhibitor of less than 5 BU. Low responders can be managed with larger quantities of FVIII concentrates. A *high responder* is defined as someone with an inhibitor of 5 to 10 BU; thus, a 10:1 mix of normal plasma with the patient's plasma that results in a 50% reduction in FVIII activity yields a BU of 10. A high responder will generate an anamnestic response to FVIII, eliminating the usefulness of FVIII replacement therapy.

Conventional treatment for hemophilia A patients with high-titer inhibitors involves the use of porcine FVIII, which is hemostatically effective in humans but sufficiently dissimilar structurally that there is little cross-reactivity with antibodies to human FVIII (Table 17.3). In the past, when porcine FVIII therapy did not work, prothrombin complex concentrates and activated prothrombin complex concentrates were used (Table 17.4). The availability of recombinant FVIIa has raised expectations that this will become the standard treatment for patients with FVIII inhibitors (see Table 17.3) (3).

There is an emerging strategy to control an inhibitor after it has developed, which is designated *immune tolerance induction*. This therapy uses large daily doses of infused human FVIII combined with immunosuppression. This treatment is given over the course of many months to years; the end point is inhibitor eradication (immune tolerance) or conversion of a high responder to a low responder. Although it is expensive and complicated, it offers the possibility of permanent inhibitor eradication. A recent economic analysis suggests that, in comparison with alternative treatment programs, immune tolerance induction may be cost-effective (4).

Factor IX Deficiency (Hemophilia B)

Hemophilia B occurs in about 1 of 30,000 male births. Over 400 individual mutations have been catalogued. Unlike hemophilia A, which is due to conserved germline mutations passed forward for over 50 generations, at least one-third of hemophilia B cases arise from new mutations in the factor IX gene at C-G dinucleotide hotspots. The FIX gene is smaller and much less complex than

Table 17.3 Replacement therapy for hemophilia patients with high-titer inhibitors

Hyate:C (Speywood)

Porcine factor VIII (used in hemophilia A only)

1 IU/kg raises plasma FVIII by 1.5 IU/dL

Measure inhibitor activity to porcine FVIII

If an inhibitor to porcine FVIII:

    Total dose = Neutralizing dose + Replacement dose

    (Neutralizing dose (IU) = Plasma volume × BU/mL; Replacement dose = Desired level − Actual level)

    Administer every 6 to 8 hours ($T_{1/2} \sim 11$ hours)

Risks: infusion reaction (4%), inhibitor worsens (rare)

Cost (wholesale): $2.20/IU

NovoSeven (Novo Nordisk)

Recombinant human factor VIIa

Administer 90 µg/kg every 2 hours until hemostasis is achieved

Risks: venous and arterial thrombosis (rare)

Cost (wholesale): $0.81/µg

Table 17.4 Factor IX products available for treatment of hemophilia B

FACTOR IX CONCENTRATES			PROTHROMBIN COMPLEX CONCENTRATES (PCCs)				ACTIVATED PCCs	
AlphaNine	Benefix	Mononine	Bebulin VH	Konyne 80	Profilnine HT	Proplex T	Autoplex	Feiba
Alpha	Genetics Institute	Centeon	Immuno	Bayer	Alpha	Baxter	Nabi	Immuno
Purified from human plasma by chromatography; solvent-detergent treated	Recombinant product with trace hamster proteins	Monoclonal antibody affinity purified, treated with sodium thiocyanate and ultrafiltered	Vapor heat-treated; contains FII, VII, IX, X	Heat-treated; contains FII, VII, IX, X	Solvent-detergent treated; contains FII, VII, IX, X	Heat-treated; contains FII, VII, IX, X	Heat-treated; contains variable amounts of activated FII, VII, IX, X	Vapor heat treated; contains FII, IX, X, and activated FVII
$T_{1/2}$ = 24 hours	$T_{1/2}$ = 24 hours	$T_{1/2}$ = 24 hours	$T_{1/2}$ = 24 hours	$T_{1/2}$ = 24 hours	$T_{1/2}$ = 24 hours	$T_{1/2}$ = 24 hours	$T_{1/2}$ = 12 hours	$T_{1/2}$ = 12 hours
1 IU/kg raises FIX level by 1.0%. Prophylactic doses are 40–80IU/kg twice per week	1 IU/kg raises FIX level by 1.0%. Prophylactic doses are 40–80IU/kg twice per week	1 IU/kg raises FIX level by 1.0%. Prophylactic doses are 40–80IU/kg twice per week	1 IU/kg raises FIX level by 1.0%; not approved for FVIII inhibitors; may cause hypercoagulable state	1 IU/kg raises FIX level by 1.0%; for FVIII inhibitors use 75 IU/kg; may cause hypercoagulable state	1 IU/kg raises FIX level by 1.0%; for FVIII inhibitors use 75 IU/kg; may cause hypercoagulable state	1 IU/kg raises FIX level by 1.0%; for FVIII inhibitors use 75 IU/kg; may cause hypercoagulable state	Dose 25–100 FVII correction units per kg every 12 hours; use only for high-titer FVIII inhibitor. *Risk for DIC and thrombosis; never use with antifibrinolytic!*	Dose 50–100 FVII correction units per kg every 12 hours; use only for high-titer FVIII inhibitor. *Risk for DIC and thrombosis; never use with antifibrinolytic!*

Abbreviations: DIC = disseminated intravascular coagulation; $T_{1/2}$ = half-life.

the FVIII gene, thereby facilitating the discovery of new mutations by whole gene sequencing techniques.

The clinical picture, diagnostic evaluation, and classification of FIX deficiency are identical to FVIII deficiency. The treatment approaches, which include using prophylactic factor IX for infants, target FIX levels, and durations of treatment (see Table 17.1), are also identical, although the types of replacement therapy for hemophilia B, and their dose and schedule, are unique (see Table 17.4). In contrast to FVIII, FIX is distributed throughout the total plasma volume with a much greater half-life. These facts translate into two practical issues: 1 IU/kg of FIX replacement raises plasma levels by only 1%, and dosing is usually done at 24 hour intervals. The cost of purified FIX is about the same as for FVIII: $1.00 to $1.20/IU wholesale price.

Replacement therapy in severe hemophilia B is complicated far less often by the development of inhibitors (<5%). However, an inhibitor to FIX can be dangerous, because it may be recognized only after a severely deficient child goes into anaphylactic shock during replacement therapy. Anaphylaxis may develop in 50% of persons with FIX inhibitor. It is more likely to occur with FIX concentrates containing other coagulation proteins. If an inhibitor is long-standing without any associated anaphylaxis and a patient requires hemostatic intervention, replacement therapy with high-dose purified FIX is recommended. If there is a history of anaphylaxis, recombinant activated FVII is the treatment of choice (see Table 17.3).

Factor XI Deficiency (Hemophilia C)

The biology of FXI is very interesting. Before its physiologic role as a coagulation system amplifier was identified (see Chapter 1), there was the conundrum of FXI deficiency. Clinical observations had noted that the level of FXI did not seem to predict clinical bleeding, spontaneous bleeding rarely occurred, and only deficient patients who were provoked or who had a personal or family history of bleeding could expect to suffer a clinically significant bleeding problem, and this could occur even when the state of deficiency was very mild. Many of these odd characteristics remain unexplained. The basis for bleeding after provocation, however, is fairly well worked out: FXI activation by small amounts of thrombin generated by the tissue factor/FVIIa pathway serves to activate FIX and the "tenase complex," thereby greatly amplifying the triggering stimulus (Chapter 1).

Factor XI deficiency is uncommon except among Ashkenazi Jews, and at least one-half of all affected persons on the planet are found in this small gene pool. Two specific mutations in the FXI gene on chromosome 4 account for over 90% of the deficiencies in the Ashkenazi population. An abnormal allele (resulting in the heterozygous state) is found in 6% to 10% of this population, and the homozygous (or mixed heterozygous) state is found in 1 out of 190 Ashkenazi living in Israel (5). Thus, the laboratory and clinical effects of FXI deficiency are perhaps best studied in this group.

The *severe* phenotype occurs with FXI levels less than 10% of normal plasma. These patients have an elevated aPTT and rarely have spontaneous bleeding, but can bleed after surgery (about 1 in 5 have excessive bleeding after gastrointestinal, gynecologic, or orthopedic surgery) or trauma. The bleeding is more common and severe following surgery on tissues that have increased local fibrinolytic activity, such as the nose, mouth, tonsils, and the genitourinary tract (where about 3 in 4 will bleed excessively). Factor XI levels over 30% usually provide adequate hemostasis, although a personal or family history of bleeding should be considered good predictors of bleeding risk in individual patients, even when their levels are nearly 50%.

Bleeding is treated with FXI replacement. This is usually provided by fresh frozen plasma (FFP) infusions, although solvent-detergent–treated plasma may soon become routinely available and may be preferred because it inactivates many viruses, including lipid envelope viruses like HIV and hepatitis viruses. A purified FXI concentrate has been used for replacement outside the United States, but its use has been associated with an unexpectedly large number of thrombotic complications; its approval by the U.S. Food and Drug Administration for use in the United States does not appear to be imminent.

The bleeding patient should receive FXI replacement sufficient to achieve a plasma level of over 40%. To prevent bleeding with surgery, prophylactic FXI is given to all patients whose FXI level is below 30%. For minor surgery, the target FXI level is 30% and it should be maintained for about 1 week. For major surgery, the target FXI level is over 45%, and it should be maintained for 7 to 10 days. For a patient with a level between 30% and 50% who gives a reliable history of bleeding (provoked or unprovoked), any treatment or prophylaxis program should aim to get the FXI level above 50%.

Standard treatment of FXI deficiency using replacement with FFP is quite simple: load with 15 mL/kg and infuse 5 mL/kg every 24 hours after loading. The half-life of FXI replaced through FFP infusions is very long (at least 2 days), so FXI measurements performed every other day often direct a decrease in the daily dose of FFP needed to maintain target FXI levels 30% to 40%. On the other hand, this empirical dose schedule is based on the assumption that FXI levels do not correlate with bleeding, and that establishing a level of 30% to 40% is adequate in most cases. If the history, surgical intent, or clinical observations indicate that more rapid and precise target FXI levels should be achieved, consider that 1 mL of FFP contains 1% FXI activity and calculate the loading dose using the standard formula:

(Target level − Baseline level) × Kg body weight = Volume of FFP required

Other Coagulation Factor Deficiencies

Deficiencies of FX, VII, V, II (prothrombin), and fibrinogen cause bleeding and an elevated aPTT. A deficiency of FXII (Hageman factor), like deficiencies of prekallikrein or high-molecular-weight kininogen, causes extreme elevations of the aPTT that challenge the most obsessive laboratory technician. None of these, however, has any effect on hemostasis. In contrast, FXIII deficiency causes severe bleeding without affecting any of the conventional coagulation tests. Congenital deficiencies or defects among the coagulation factors presented in Table 17.5 are very rare, but acquired combined deficiencies of fibrinogen, FII, FV, FVII, and FX from liver disease and/or vitamin K deficiency are common (see Chapter 19). FX deficiency is also associated with amyloidosis because amyloid deposits bind and sequester FX. The information in Table 17.5 applies equally to both congenital and acquired deficiencies, although acquired disorders *never cause an absolute deficiency.*

A mixing study to rule out an inhibitor is an essential step in evaluating a patient with a suspected deficiency of one of the coagulation factors in Table 17.5. This is important because there are nearly as many reported cases of inhibitors to these factors as there are inherited deficiencies, and treatments for a factor inhibitor are different from those treatments listed below (see Chapter 18).

The Horizon: Gene Therapy

Many safe products are available to treat patients with hemophilia. Prophylactic factor programs hold out the promise of giving severe hemophiliacs the opportunity to return to normal lifestyles and full life spans. No hemophiliac has been infected with HIV since 1987. The current pasteurization and solvent/detergent viral inactivation processes remove all viruses except parvovirus and hepatitis A. The former infection is considered clinically trivial and the latter infection is almost eliminated by the donor screening process (see Chapter 13). Nonetheless, there will always be anxiety about a new pathogen that escapes both the collection screen and all viral inactivation procedures. There is great concern and debate about the possibility of transmitting a prion-borne disease through the use of products derived from human blood (6). In response to this concern, recombinant products that contain no human blood products (albumin-free) are entering the market. Recombinant FVIII and FIX genetically engineered to improve pharmacokinetics and therapeutic index are imminent. With so many amazing successes sweeping the field, it is reasonable to ask where gene therapy fits into the future of hemophilia care.

The prophylaxis programs have made it evident to the hemophilia community that tiny increases in plasma factor levels could have a major impact on disease-related morbidity. Thus, the promise of gene therapy for hemophilia will be realized when factor levels are restored to over 5% (mild hemophilia), but important clinical benefits could be gained even by converting a severe hemophiliac into a moderate hemophiliac (factor level of little more than 1%). The technical achievements required to achieve a factor level of 1% safely and comfortably will be overcome sooner or later.

At this time there are several active phase 1 clinical trials of gene therapy for both hemophilia B and hemophilia A. The next decade not only should establish the feasibility of gene therapy for hemophilia, but will define its therapeutic

Table 17.5 Rare coagulation deficiencies

	FIBRINOGEN DEFICIENCY	PROTHROMBIN DEFICIENCY	FACTOR V DEFICIENCY	FACTOR VII DEFICIENCY	FACTOR X DEFICIENCY	FACTOR XII DEFICIENCY	FACTOR XIII DEFICIENCY
	Umbilical, intracranial, GI, mucosal, and menstrual bleeding; hemarthrosis in 20%; pregnancy complications	Life-long mild–moderate bleeding; no hemarthrosis	Mild-severe bleeding; including hemarthrosis; 50% affected develop problems as adults	Severe bleeding when level <1%; variable expression with FVII 1–10%; provoked bleeding with levels 10%–25%	Severe bleeding when level <1%; variable expression with FX 1–10%; provoked bleeding with levels 10–15%	No bleeding	When level <1%: umbilical stump bleeding, hematomas, hemarthroses, intracranial bleeding (25%), delayed bleeding, poor wound healing, miscarriages
	Quantitative and qualitative disorders	Quantitative	Quantitative	Quantitative	Quantitative	Quantitative	Quantitative
	Autosomal recessive; many mutations on chromosome 4	Autosomal recessive; gene on chromosome 11	Autosomal recessive; gene on chromosome 1	Autosomal recessive; gene on chromosome 13	Autosomal recessive; gene on chromosome 13	Autosomal recessive; gene on chromosome 5	Autosomal recessive; gene on chromosome 6
	PT, aPTT, and thrombin time ↑↑ (heterozygotes) to ∞ (homozygotes); fibrinogen measured functionally and by protein assay; when these tests are disparate, consider dysfibrinogenemia.	↑ PT and aPTT	↑ PT and aPTT	↑↑ PT; aPTT normal	↑ PT; aPTT ↑ or normal	aPTT ↑↑ (heterozygotes) aPTT ∞ (homozygotes)	PT, aPTT, and thrombin time are normal; clots lyse in 5 Molar urea within minutes (versus 24 hours for normal clots).

~200 cases of congenital hypo- and afibrinogenemia, and ~200 cases of congenital dysfibrinogenemia, worldwide.	<50 cases	~150 cases	Rare congenital but common acquired disorder	Rare	Several hundred cases	>100 cases
In afibrinogenemic persons who are bleeding or undergoing elective surgery: replace with cryoprecipitate, which contains ~250 mg fibrinogen/unit. Treat with a dose of 4 bags/10 kg (each bag contains ~10 units) and repeat 2 bags/10 kg every 48 hours as needed. $T_{1/2}$ = 90 hours.	FFP targeted to a FII level of 25%: 15–20 mL/kg followed by 5 mL/kg every 24 hours. $T_{1/2}$ = 72 hours; prothrombin complex concentrates can also be used when FFP fails.	FFP targeted to a FV level of 20%: 15–20 mL/kg followed by 5 mL/kg every 24 hours. $T_{1/2}$ = 36 hours.	FFP targeted to a FVII level of 20%: 15–20 mL/kg followed by 5 mL/kg every 6–12 hours. $T_{1/2}$ = 6 hours; prothrombin complex concentrates can also be used when FFP fails.	FFP targeted to a FX level of 20%: 15–20 mL/kg followed by 5 mL/kg every 24 hours. $T_{1/2}$ = 40 hours; prothrombin complex concentrates can also be used when FFP fails.	No treatment. May lead to increased risk of venous thrombosis because FXII catalyzes the conversion of plasminogen to plasmin.	FXIII = "fibrin stabilizing factor." It is a transglutaminase that cross-links fibrin polymers. Replacement with small amounts of FFP (2–3 mL/kg) or cryoprecipitate (1 bag/10 kg) is effective. Give monthly. $T_{1/2}$ = 2 weeks.

Abbreviations: aPPT = activated partial thromboplastin time; FFP = fresh frozen plasma; GI = gastrointestinal; PT = prothrombin time; $T_{1/2}$ = half-life.

index, compare clinical outcomes between different treatment programs, and measure its cost-effectiveness (7). Every advance along these lines of research will fan out into other areas of clinical investigation and benefit humans in ways that are currently only barely imaginable.

Annotated Bibliography

1. Soucie JM, Nuss R, Evatt B, et al. Mortality among males living with hemophilia: relations with source of medical care. The Hemophilia Surveillance System Project. Blood 2000;96:422–437.

   This study evaluated 2950 patients for an average of 2.6 years. In this group, the age-adjusted mortality was 40 deaths per 1000 persons per year, primarily from AIDS and hepatitis virus–induced liver disease. As can be inferred from the report's title, survival was significantly greater among persons cared for by comprehensive hemophilia treatment centers.

2. Ljung RCR. Prophylactic infusion regimens in the management of hemophilia. Thromb Haemost 1999;82:525–530.

   A must-read for everyone interested in hemophilia. This paper reviews the practical experience of implementing WHO recommendations to provide prophylaxis for all children with severe hemophilia A. Although the situation provides an outstanding opportunity for the medical and scientific community to do the right thing, a comparison with President Richard M. Nixon's "war on cancer" is inevitable: public opinion and political charges (both uninformed) neglect to consider the state of science and economics. Often recommendations are easier said than done—but when they are done, they will be an achievement of historic proportions.

3. Hedner U. Treatment of patients with factor VIII and factor IX inhibitors with special focus on the use of recombinant factor VIIa. Thromb Haemost 1999;82:531–539.

   A thorough review of the therapeutic index of all treatments available for hemophiliacs with inhibitors.

4. Colowick AB, Bohn RL, Avorn J, Ewenstein BM. Immune tolerance induction in hemophilia patients with inhibitors: costly can be cheaper. Blood 2000;96:1698–1702.

   A decision-analytic model was applied to investigating the overall costs of immune tolerance induction (ITI). The cost of ITI for a 5 year old is estimated at about $1 million. Over that child's lifetime, which is estimated to increase by about 5 years as a result of ITI, the protocol would save the health care system almost $2 million. To quote Dr. Seuss, "What would *you* do?"

5. Asakai R, Chung DW, Davie EW, Seligsohn U. Factor XI deficiency in Ashkenazi Jews in Israel. N Eng J Med 1991;325:153–158.

   This study examined 43 patients. Of 86 alleles, 42 contained a Glu → Stop mutation at codon 117 and 40 contained a Phe → Leu mutation at residue

283. Both the homozygotes and the compound heterozygotes had elevated aPTTs, FXI levels below 10%, and a bleeding disorder, particularly during surgery of the urinary tract or tooth extraction. The heterozygotes had normal aPTTs and factor levels with mean values above 50%. Bleeding was not reported among the heterozygotes.

6. Drohan WN, Cervenakova L. Safety of blood products: are transmissible spongiform encephalopathies (prion diseases) a risk? Thromb Haemost 1999;82:486–493.

A detailed analysis of the present state of information about prion diseases in humans and the likelihood that they will get into the blood supply, evade detection, and resist current viral inactivation processes. Very little is known, in fact, although "a number of factors all point to a negligible risk of a person developing Creutzfeldt-Jakob disease." These factors are 1) a low prevalence of CJD in the general population, 2) no epidemiologic data that CJD is blood-related, 3) low or absent infectivity of blood from CJD patients, and 4) low efficiency of intravenous transmission to experimental animals. Also, most of the prion protein is removed from blood that has been spiked with prions when the blood is subjected to standard fractionation procedures.

7. Lusher JM. Gene therapy for hemophilia A and B: patient selection and follow-up, requirements for a cure. Thromb Haemost 1999;82:572–575.

A concise explanation of what gene therapy for hemophilia is all about. A broad outline of the goals, risks, and several incremental benefits that will be derived from gene therapy bench research and clinical trials.

18

Coagulation Factor Inhibitors

Clinical Overview

The previous chapter describes inhibitors to factor VIII (FVIII) and FIX that arise as a consequence of alloantibodies generated when replacement therapy exposes a severe hemophiliac to a "foreign protein" (the deficient coagulation factor). Coagulation factor inhibitors can also arise de novo to create an autoimmune coagulopathy (1). The most common of these are anti-FVIII antibodies, but autoantibodies can affect the activity of all coagulation proteins. The clinical approach to coagulation factor inhibitors is a hybrid between approaches used for FVIII inhibitors in patients with hemophilia and approaches used for patients with nonhematological autoimmune diseases. Coagulation factor inhibitors are rare but their clinical impact can be devastating, so it is important to recognize and treat them quickly.

Risks for the Development of Coagulation Factor Inhibitors

Most spontaneous coagulation factor inhibitors occur in older patients. There is no gender predilection. FVIII inhibitors are usually oligoclonal and idiopathic, but the association between a FVIII inhibitor and lupus, rheumatoid arthritis, solid tumors, drug reactions, and asthma has been reported. There is also a distinct syndrome of postpartum FVIII inhibitors (2,3). Polyclonal antibodies to FV are the next most common spontaneous inhibitors affecting hemostasis. They develop during the postoperative period in almost two-thirds of cases, and are probably related to the use of topical bovine thrombin and/or fibrin glues. Topical bovine thrombin can also lead to sensitization resulting in the polyclonal generation of antibodies that cross-react with endogenous prothrombin (FII) and thrombin. Factor V inhibitors also are reported to develop after exposure to aminoglycoside antibiotics and blood transfusions, and in association with solid tumors.

Most of the other inhibitors are so rare that there are few data to permit generalizations about etiological factors and pathogenesis except to state that lymphoproliferative and plasma cell disorders are probably the most common conditions in which to find an inhibitor of any type. Pathophysiological factors unique to specific inhibitors are discussed in this chapter.

Diagnosis

The clinical presentation from autoantibodies to FVIII is usually a severe bleeding disorder manifested by intractable mucosa bleeding, deep muscle bleeding (including compartment hematomas that threaten limb blood supply), and life-threatening hemodynamic compromise. Over 80% of those affected by an inhibitor to FVIII have major bleeding and over 20% of those affected die as a complication of the FVIII inhibitor. In contrast, bleeding from FV inhibitors is less common and severe bleeding is distinctly uncommon. The reason for this is that platelets contain FV in their alpha granules and secrete it when they are activated. This platelet pool of FV is resistant to the effects of anti-FV antibodies. These observations form the rationale for using platelet transfusions to treat severe bleeding associated with an inhibitor to FV (see below). The magnitude of the bleeding diathesis with other inhibitors is not predictable: everything from asymptomatic cases to cases of deadly bleeding has been reported.

Laboratory testing reveals an elevated PT and/or aPTT that doesn't correct with mixing. Two considerations direct the mixing study. First, it is essential that a heparin effect is excluded, and this can be done by mixing the specimen of blood with a heparin-binding resin. Second, the heterogeneity of antibodies to coagulation factors forces one to always consider a low titer or low avidity inhibitor that can be overcome immediately after mixing but gradually affects the activity of its target coagulation factor during a prolonged mixed incubation reaction. The diagnostic test in these cases is a mixed aPTT or PT that corrects immediately but then elevates over the course of 1 to 2 hours.

Following the determination that the elevated aPTT and/or PT is due to an inhibitor, the next step is to rule out a lupus anticoagulant by demonstrating that the elevated aPTT and/or PT (with a lupus inhibitor it is usually an elevated aPTT) does *not* correct when phospholipid or platelets are added to the reaction (see Chapter 9).

When a non-lupus inhibitor is diagnosed, the next step is to identify the affected factor by direct activity measurements of those factors most likely affected. A FVIII inhibitor is most common and causes only aPTT elevation. The next most common inhibitor is directed against FV, and this usually results in an elevated PT and aPTT. A more broadly reacting inhibitor is a prothrombin inhibitor that elevates both the PT and aPTT, but also typically cross-reacts with thrombin and causes the thrombin time to be elevated.

The final step in evaluating a spontaneous coagulation factor inhibitor is to establish its potency in Bethesda units (BU), defined as the reciprocal of the dilution of the affected person's plasma that causes a 50% reduction in the activity of the target coagulation factor in a mixing study. For example, if 50% activity results from a 1:1 mix (normal plasma/patient's plasma) it is 1 BU; if

50% activity results from a 20:1 mix (normal plasma/patient's plasma) it is 20 BU.

Management

Factor VIII inhibitors are the most commonly identified of all coagulation factor inhibitors. Treatment for them has been reasonably fine-tuned, based primarily on the perspective of Northwestern University's Dr. David Green (Table 18.1). He suggests a management algorithm based on the intensity of the inhibitor (1).

These algorithms are derived empirically. Their use requires frequent measurements of inhibitor activity (aPTT and FVIII levels) and intensive clinical monitoring. The basis for the use of porcine FVIII (Hyate:C) is that most anti-human FVIII antibodies cross-react only weakly with pig FVIII. A loading dose is administered to try to bind up by adsorption as much of the circulating inhibitor as possible. Another trick to consider is using FVIII concentrates that contain von Willebrand factor (Humate-P), which in some cases protects FVIII against the inhibitory effects of very tight antibody binding.

With FVIII and FVIIa treatments, there is some evidence that a clinical response is inevitable as long as the dose is pushed high enough. This point of view must be balanced by the belief that there is an increased risk of thrombosis as the dosage of these agents escalates. In fact, the risk of thrombosis limits the dosage of activated prothrombin complex concentrates (see Chapter 17) to an upper limit of around 100 IU/kg.

Treatment directed against the antibody begins with oral prednisone. A good response, defined as a rise in FVIII by 20% (20 IU/dL = 0.2 IU/mL) and the cessation of bleeding, occurs in about 30% of patients. In these cases, prednisone is continued until the inhibitor resolves, with dose tapering as the clinical and

Table 18.1   Algorithm for managing factor VIII inhibitors

• All patients
Prednisone 1 mg/kg/day
• Less than 5 BU without limb- or life-threatening bleeding
Desmopressin 0.3 μg/kg. If no response → Recombinant human FVIII 100 IU/kg, then 10 IU/kg/hour[a] → Porcine FVIII 50–100 IU/kg then 4 IU/kg/hour
• 5–10 BU with serious limb- or life-threatening bleeding
Porcine FVIII 50–100 IU/kg then 4 IU/kg/hour → Recombinant FVIIa 90 μg/kg every 2–3 hours[a] *or* Activated prothrombin complex concentrate 50–75 IU/kg every 8–12 hours
• >30 BU with serious limb- or life-threatening bleeding
Porcine FVIII 100–200 IU/kg then 10 IU/kg/hour[a] → Recombinant FVIIa 90 μg/kg every 2–3 hours *or* Activated prothrombin complex concentrate 50–100 IU/kg every 8–12 hours

Abbreviation: BU = Bethesda units.

[a] Can be preceded by plasmapheresis or protein A column immunoadsorption.

laboratory measurements dictate. If there is no response within 3 weeks, daily oral cyclophosphamide (2 mg/kg) is given for 3 to 6 weeks (without or with prednisone). If this fails, one can use an immune tolerance induction-like program (see Chapter 17), combination chemotherapy (like cyclophosphamide, vincristine, and prednisone), or cyclosporine (5 mg/kg/day to achieve blood levels between 150 and 350 ng/mL). High dose intravenous immunoglobulin (1 g/kg/day for 2 days) may reduce the inhibitor titer in up to 20% of patients. Plasmapheresis or immunoadsorption with a protein A column have also been used successfully to reduce the level of coagulation factor inhibitors. These last three interventions usually are transitory and must be repeated at intervals determined by the clinical and laboratory pictures. The natural history of an acquired FVIII inhibitor involves spontaneous resolution in about a third of patients, but the timeframe of resolution is sometimes years.

Postpartum factor VIII inhibitors are rare, but they present a unique clinical syndrome. They usually develop within 3 months of delivery, but prepartum cases of FVIII inhibitors have been reported and some FVIII inhibitors do not emerge until nearly a year has passed since parturition (2,3). Postpartum FVIII inhibitors usually develop in primiparous women. Treatments are similar to those outlined above, except that steroid responses are rare and some practitioners recommend immediate therapy with cyclophosphamide. About 30% resolve within 1 year, and most resolve within 3 years. Maternal and fetal mortality are low as long as intensive replacement and immune suppression therapy are implemented rapidly. Among women whose postpartum FVIII inhibitors resolve, recurrences with subsequent pregnancies are rare.

Factor V inhibitors are usually temporally associated with an operation, particularly surgery employing topical bovine thrombin or fibrin glues, both of which are contaminated with bovine FV that causes an immune response cross-reacting with endogenous FV. They typically develop in older patients within a few weeks of surgery. In the postoperative setting they tend to be ephemeral, lasting only a few months. Severe bleeding is rare. Bleeding and its prevention are usually managed with platelet transfusions because platelets supply antibody-resistant FV to sites of hemostatic need. Plasmapheresis is the best way to accomplish antibody removal, which may be necessary for patients who develop an autoantibody to FV de novo (about 20% of cases). Steroids and cytotoxic agent–mediated immunosuppression tend not to work with FV inhibitors.

Spontaneous acquired thrombin, factor II, VII, IX, X, XI, XII, XIII, and fibrin inhibitors are extremely uncommon. In general, the antibody is treated with immunosuppression (prednisone and/or cyclophosphamide) and plasmapheresis. Antifibrinolytic therapy can be tried in all cases (except those receiving activated prothrombin complex concentrates) and in some cases it works to control bleeding. Otherwise, replacement therapy directed toward the specific coagulation factor deficiency is used for bleeding. As stated above, antibodies to **thrombin** and/or **prothrombin** can follow the use of topical thrombin or fibrin sealant. In addition, heparin-like molecules that inhibit thrombin have been observed in patients with myeloma and transitional cell carcinoma, and in patients on hemodialysis or persons receiving the antineoplastic drug suramin.

Protamine can be used to treat bleeding when the thrombin inhibitor is a heparin-like molecule (see Chapter 5). **Factor VII inhibitors** lead to an isolated PT. The few cases that have been reported had very severe bleeding. Treatment with recombinant FVIIa is recommended. Spontaneous **FIX inhibitors** are treated with large doses of FIX concentrates (to adsorb the antibody) followed by activated prothrombin complex concentrates. If these measures fail, recombinant FVIIa is recommended. Factor X autoantibodies are reportedly short-lived and not associated with severe bleeding. If severe bleeding from a **FX inhibitor** occurs it is treated with fresh frozen plasma (FFP) or prothrombin complex concentrates. **Factor XI inhibitors** can also be treated with FFP. Inhibitors of fibrinogen cleavage or fibrin polymerization are usually associated with multiple myeloma or Waldenström's macroglobulinemia and their treatment targets the underlying disease.

Finally, **inhibitors to FXIII** can occur. It is interesting to note that they sometimes arise associated with isoniazid (INH) therapy for mycobacterial diseases. INH reacts directly with FXIII and alters its structure to the point of creating new epitopes that trigger an immune response. FXIII inhibitors are often lethal (over one-quarter of cases in one series resulted in death). Bleeding associated with FXIII inhibitors is best treated with large doses of cryoprecipitate (or a FXIII concentrate if it is available).

Annotated Bibliography

1. Feinstein DI, Green D, Federici AB, Goodnight SH Jr. Diagnosis and management of patients with spontaneously acquired inhibitors of coagulation. Hematology 1999: American Society of Hematology education book. Washington, 1999: American Society of Hematology, 1999:192–208. (Also available at http//:www.hematology.org.)

   This chapter covers antiphospholipid antibodies, the acquired von Willebrand syndrome and all coagulation factor inhibitors. It provides several useful tables about clinical, laboratory, and treatment approaches for factor VIII inhibitors.

2. Hauser I, Schneider B, Lechner K. Postpartum factor VIII inhibitors. A review of the literature with special reference to the value of steroid and immunosuppressive treatment. Thromb Haemost 1995;73:1–5.

3. Solymoss S. Postpartum acquired factor VIII inhibitors: results of a survey. Am J Hematol 1998;59:1–4.

   These two references describe 65 cases of postpartum FVIII inhibitors. The general pattern is a primiparous woman who starts bleeding after she has been discharged from the hospital. The bleeding can be very severe and is manageable with routine replacement therapy, including recombinant FVIIa. Immunosuppression is perhaps most effectively achieved with oral cyclophosphamide. Fetal and maternal mortality are very low with intensive supportive care and immunosuppression.

19

Acquired Coagulopathies

The consultant is often invited to assist in managing coagulation disturbances that develop among patients who have similar risks related to similar problems. Lumping patients into groups based on a shared clinical problem leading to shared hemostatic challenges can streamline the bedside approach that one takes when evaluating a patient with serious clinical bleeding, and can simplify the development of a differential diagnosis and the implementation of a treatment plan. This chapter addresses certain clinical conditions that are commonly encountered and are associated with a set of predictable coagulation disturbances.

The Surgical Patient

Anticoagulant management in surgical patients involves two issues: 1) how to organize chronic warfarin anticoagulation during the perioperative period, and 2) how to organize the initiation of anticoagulation therapy for patients after the surgery. Table 19.1 gives recommendations about how to manage chronic anticoagulation (1). There are several interesting clinical points that relate to these recommendations.

First, it takes about 4 days for an INR of 2.0–3.0 to reach 1.5 after warfarin is stopped, and all surgery except elective spine and brain surgery can be performed safely at that point (all coagulation abnormalities should be reversed whenever possible when spine or brain surgery is being done).

Second, the risk of recurrence is always greatest nearest to the thrombotic event, and major surgery within 4 weeks of an acute thrombosis should be avoided if possible. If postponing surgery is not an option and the thrombotic event is a deep venous thrombosis (DVT) or pulmonary embolism (PE) less than 2 weeks old, an IVC filter should be placed because the risk of bleeding with anticoagulation is high and anticoagulant therapy interruption (usually for 6 hours preoperatively, plus the duration of the operation, plus 12 hours postoperatively) is estimated to result in about a 2% risk of recurrence during the treatment hiatus. If surgery is performed within 3 to 4 weeks of the acute throm-

Table 19.1   **Anticoagulant therapy in surgical patients**

CLINICAL SETTING	PREOPERATIVELY	POSTOPERATIVELY
Acute venous thromboembolism (VTE)		
Within 2 weeks	IVC filter	IVC filter
Within 2–4 weeks	Intravenous heparin stopped 6 hours before surgery	Intravenous heparin (1000 U/hour) started 12 hours after surgery
After 4 weeks	Stop warfarin for 3 to 4 days (INR < 1.5)	Intravenous heparin (1000 U/hour) started 12 hours after surgery
Recurrent VTE	Stop warfarin for 3–4 days (INR < 1.5)	Subcutaneous heparin (e.g., 5000 U, twice a day) or low-molecular-weight heparin (e.g., 30 mg twice a day), started 12 hours after surgery
Acute arterial thrombosis within 1 month	Intravenous heparin stopped 6 hours before surgery	Intravenous heparin (1000 U/hour) started 12 hours after surgery
Mechanical heart valve	Stop warfarin for 3 to 4 days (INR < 1.5)	Subcutaneous heparin (e.g., 5000 U, twice a day) or low-molecular-weight heparin (e.g., 30 mg, twice a day) started 12 hours after surgery
Chronic atrial fibrillation	Stop warfarin for 3 to 4 days (INR < 1.5)	Subcutaneous heparin (e.g., 5000 U, twice a day) or low-molecular-weight heparin (e.g., 30 mg, twice a day) started 12 hours after surgery

bosis, the patient requires a heparin infusion that is stopped 6 hours preoperatively and restarted 12 postoperatively.

Third, postoperative management *always* aims to start heparin 12 hours postoperatively. However, if the patient is bleeding, the heparin should be delayed or an IVC filter placed. If the patient is at an increased risk for thrombosis and full heparin anticoagulation is required (see Table 19.1), restart the 1000 U/hour heparin infusion without a bolus. Use a heparin infusion whenever the risk of bleeding is high, even if the dose is at the lower "prophylactic" level, so that the heparin can be turned off immediately if bleeding starts.

Finally, heparin is used until warfarin anticoagulation returns the INR to >2.0. Warfarin is restarted at 5 mg per day within a few days of the operation, depending on the postoperative course and the bedside assessment of bleeding risk.

Postoperative prophylactic anticoagulation therapy is usually started as per the usual routines described in Chapter 4. In most cases these methods are associated with an acceptably low risk of bleeding (<5% major bleeding) with a large decrease in risk of thrombosis (>50% in most cases). A patient who is bleeding must receive prophylaxis, but it should be nonpharmacologic prophylaxis. The most intensive form of nonpharmacologic prophylaxis is intermittent pneumatic compression. This method is safe and effective, although there is no evidence that it is as good as routine pharmacologic prophylaxis. Graduated compression stockings (like "TED" stockings) are also effective at decreasing the risk of DVT (although perhaps not PE), perhaps equal to pharmacologic intervention in moderate risk patients (about 60% reduction). Both of these devices should be started before surgery, continued through surgery, and worn until ambulation returns. Graduated compression stockings are recommended generally for all patients except those with leg artery insufficiency. They enhance the effectiveness of intermittent pneumatic compression and pharmacological prophylaxis, and decrease the complications of postphlebitic syndrome in venous thromboembolism (VTE) patients.

Neurosurgical and spinal cord surgery patients require special consideration. Prophylaxis in neurosurgery is best accomplished with a combination of low-molecular-weight heparin (LMWH) plus graduated compression stockings (see the references for Chapter 4). Nonpharmacologic methods are recommended for spinal cord surgery patients, as well as for brain injury and spinal cord trauma patients. These situations can be made much worse by anticoagulant therapy, and therefore the best interventions for VTE are intermittent pneumatic compression for prevention and an IVC filter for treatment.

The final issue to consider is the optimal **VTE prophylaxis of a patient who is receiving anesthesia through an epidural catheter.** Epidural catheters may remain in place for several days and there have been episodes of cord compression from spinal hematomas among patients receiving prophylactic heparin. The current recommendations are

1. Use 40 mg of subcutaneous enoxaparin each day as VTE prophylaxis.
2. Place the catheter at least 12 hours after the dose of enoxaparin.
3. Resume enoxaparin no sooner than 2 hours after catheter placement.
4. Remove the catheter no sooner than 12 to 24 hours after the last enoxaparin injection.
5. Do not restart enoxaparin for at least 2 hours after catheter removal.
6. All other antihemostatic drugs must be avoided in these patients.

The Obstetrical Patient

Pregnancy is associated with several expected coagulation disturbances. These include the ubiquitous, transient pregnancy–associated hypercoagulable state (Chapter 10) and incidental thrombocytopenia (Chapter 14). Pregnancy confounds the routine management of VTE (Chapter 4) and immune thrombocytopenias (ITP, Chapter 14), and creates a unique setting for several common (preeclampsia, eclampsia, and HELLP syndrome; see Chapter 14) and uncommon (neonatal immune thrombocytopenia; see Chapter 14) coagulation disturbances. Pregnancy is also associated with several complications that lead to a very unstable state of coagulation that can culminate in a catastrophic outcome, such as abruptio placentae, intrauterine fetal demise, and amniotic fluid embolism. Finally, there is increasing evidence that recurrent miscarriages and other unfavorable gestational and perhaps maternal (separate from VTE) outcomes are related to unrecognized inherited hypercoagulable factors in the mother.

The routine management of VTE during pregnancy must avoid warfarin, which is teratogenic. Although LMWH has never been compared to unfractionated heparin in pregnant women, it has emerged as the treatment of choice because it is easier and less often associated with heparin-induced thrombocytopenia and osteoporosis. For acute treatment, 1 mg/kg of enoxaparin, twice a day, is given for 7 to 10 days. For maintenance treatment following an acute VTE, or for chronically anticoagulated women, or for prophylaxis or treatment of at risk pregnancies (see below), 40 mg of enoxaparin every day is recommended. During the last trimester subcutaneous injections should be administered into the upper legs. LMWH should be continued for 6 weeks postpartum. The importance of VTE prevention and treatment in pregnant women cannot be overemphasized: *pulmonary embolism is the leading cause of maternal death in the United States*. A recent study indicates that it is safe to withhold heparin from pregnant women who have a history of VTE, but postpartum anticoagulation for 4 to 6 weeks should be administered (2).

Abruptio placentae is the premature separation of the placenta from the uterus. It may arise as a consequence of placental vessel ischemia/infarction due to an inherited thrombophilia, and it may result in disseminated intravascular coagulation (DIC). Abruptio placentae is treated with immediate delivery. Depending on the magnitude of DIC and its associated coagulation abnormalities, delivery can be supported with platelets, fresh frozen plasma, and cryoprecipitate. Heparin should never be used for this condition.

Intrauterine fetal demise can also lead to DIC. It is a rare event that only occurs after the 20th week of gestation and only if the dead fetus is retained for several weeks. Treatment requires fetus removal. If DIC is life threatening, full-dose unfractionated heparin has been used successfully in conjunction with blood products and fetal delivery.

Amniotic fluid embolism is a tragic complication of an otherwise normal pregnancy and parturition. It occurs rarely (1 in 40,000 deliveries). It is usually fatal, accounting for 10% of all the maternal deaths in the United States. About 70% occur during vaginal deliveries. Affected women suffer acute cardiopulmonary collapse and their undelivered child develops intrauterine distress. There is a registry collecting cases of amniotic fluid embolism (see Am J Obstet Gynecol 1995; 172: 1158). Criteria for registration are 1) acute hypotension or cardiac arrest, 2) acute hypoxia (dyspnea, cyanosis, or respiratory arrest), 3) coagulopathy, 4) onset of the above during labor, cesarian section, or dilation and evacuation, or within 20 minutes of delivery, and 5) no other conditions that account for the signs and symptoms observed. The cause of amniotic fluid embolism is unknown. Treatment is supportive care, which almost always involves intensive blood product support, including cryoprecipitate for severe hypofibrinogenemia.

Recurrent miscarriages affect 2% of women. Besides the antiphospholipid antibody syndrome (APS) (see Chapter 9), several other hypercoagulable states appear to increase the risk of recurrent miscarriages. The mechanism by which a hypercoagulable state leads to miscarriage is uncertain, but placental vascular thrombosis is believed to be the common denominator. In addition to miscarriage, placental ischemia or infarction from thrombosis is probably associated with intrauterine fetal demise, preeclampsia, the HELLP syndrome (hemolysis with elevated liver function tests and low platelets), and abruptio placentae (3). It is therefore reasonable to look for a hypercoagulable state beyond the APS as a cause for these conditions as well as recurrent fetal loss. The evaluation should start with testing for factor V Leiden, activated protein C resistance, prothrombin G20210A, or antithrombin (AT) III deficiency. If these are not present, then one can investigate for low levels of protein C, protein S, hyperhomocystinemia, or dysfibrinogenemia. If an antiphospholipid antibody, factor V Leiden, deficiency of protein C or S, prothrombin G20210A, or a combination of defects is discovered, an affected woman can be treated with low-molecular-weight heparin throughout pregnancy up to the time of delivery. For example, any of these conditions except the APS could be treated with enoxaparin at a prophylactic dose of 30 mg subcutaneously twice a day. For APS, the dose of enoxaparin is 30–40 mg subcutaneously once a day. The decision to treat must take into consideration that presently there are no clinical data that anticoagulant therapy is predictably effective in preventing unfavorable pregnancy outcomes in any condition except APS.

The Infected Patient

Bacteremia is associated with transient isolated thrombocytopenia that can be quite severe (4). It is caused by nonspecific adsorption of opsonized bacteria and antibodies to platelets, resulting in splenic clearance. Bacteremia resulting in the syndrome of **sepsis** causes DIC. This is particularly common in gram-negative bacteremia (30% to 50% have associated DIC).

Certain **antibiotics** affect platelet numbers and functions (see Chapters 14 and 15). One must also be aware that infection can indirectly lead to vitamin K deficiency. The intensive care unit patient who is not eating and is receiving several antibiotics is the person most likely to develop **vitamin K deficiency**. The body's store of vitamin K is only good for about 1 week. Without dietary intake, commensal intestinal flora make enough vitamin K to maintain the synthesis of factors II, VII, IX, and X day to day, but when these bacteria are hindered by antibiotics, the total body vitamin K stores fall abruptly to almost zero. Vitamin K deficiency causes an elevation of the PT that corrects with mixing. Measurement of FV and FVII distinguishes the coagulopathies of vitamin K deficiency and liver disease (both are decreased in liver disease). Treatment with 10 mg of parenteral vitamin K reverses this coagulopathy.

The Heart Attack Patient

Patients with unstable angina and myocardial infarction are susceptible to bleeding from medications used to paralyze the hemostatic system. These medications include heparin or hirudin, platelet GpIIb-IIIa blockers, thrombolytic therapy, aspirin, or ticlopidine/clopidogrel (see Chapter 6). Treatment for clinically significant bleeding must first involve ranking the therapeutic index of each agent. The next step is to stop the most likely cause of the bleeding. Finally, based on the pharmacokinetics of the putative offending agent, the patient must simply be supported until the hemorrhagic complications resolve spontaneously or some action must be taken to reverse the hemostatic disturbance. Infusions of heparin, hirudin, or thrombolytics present systemic levels of medications with a very short half-life, so stopping them is usually sufficient to halt bleeding. When stopping the infusion is not enough, various additional measures can be employed to reverse the hemostatic imbalance (see Chapters 5, 7, 8, and 14).

Parenteral antiplatelet agents will affect platelets for a day or two after they are stopped, and bleeding attributed to them should be treated with platelet transfusions.

Impaired hemostasis is the *sine qua non* of modern treatments for coronary artery disease, and clinically mild to moderate bleeding must sometimes be tolerated to preserve blood flow to the at-risk myocardium.

The Patient with Cancer

Patients with **solid tumors** are vulnerable to venous thromboembolism and migratory superficial thrombophlebitis. Cancer, both directly and indirectly, causes hypercoagulability by affecting the venous circuit. VTE can sometimes be the first evidence of a solid tumor, and almost 15% of new VTEs are associated with cancer (5) (see Chapter 10, reference 10).

A routine workup at presentation is adequate to identify the cancer, which is usually evident within 6 months of the VTE. The cancer is at an advanced and incurable stage in about one-half of all cases. VTE is *not* a cancer warning sign that directs one to an occult early stage cancer that is curable by surgery. The most common cancers associated with VTE—pancreas, ovary, hepatocellular, and brain—are notoriously difficult to treat in advanced stages.

Trousseau's syndrome is a migratory superficial thrombophlebitis in which the inflammatory component of the disease process (particularly pain and redness) is clinically vexing. It most often develops in association with mucin-producing adenocarcinomas of the gastrointestinal tract or prostate because mucin directly activates the intrinsic coagulation system. But any patient with any solid tumor can develop Trousseau's syndrome, probably because any cancer can at some point synthesize tissue factor. Trousseau's syndrome almost always accompanies advanced cancer, for which treatments are limited, so chemotherapy or radiotherapy to reverse the underlying disease process is not usually effective against it.

Treatment with heparin anticoagulants and/or recombinant antithrombin III sometimes palliates the symptoms. Warfarin is probably contraindicated because of frequent bleeding side effects. Heparin is administered based on the principle of trial and error. Unfractionated heparin or LMWH has been tried at very low doses and at very high doses; the only measure of good dosing is decreased symptoms without significant bleeding.

Trousseau's syndrome is often associated with laboratory abnormalities of low-grade DIC, including deficient plasma ATIII concentration. Because of the acquired ATIII deficiency and the consistent clinical observations that Trousseau's syndrome is notoriously refractory to heparin, ATIII concentrates have been used alone and with heparin to treat the symptoms; sometimes patients respond to ATIII infusions (see Chapter 10 for dosing program). In some situations, pharmacologic doses rather than "replacement" doses of ATIII work.

Chemotherapy can affect the coagulation system. The most consistent coagulopathy triggered by chemotherapy is the hypofibrinogenemia or dysfibrinogenemia caused by the direct effect of L-asparaginase, used to treat acute lymphocytic leukemia, on hepatic synthesis of fibrinogen. This can lead to bleeding or to a DIC-like state associated with thrombosis. Actinomycin inhibits the gamma carboxylation of factors II, VII, IX, and X. Mitomycin is associated with a microangiopathic hemolytic anemia. Mithramycin, which is used more often for hypercalcemia associated with malignancy rather than as an antineoplastic drug, induces a qualitative platelet abnormality that causes bleeding in almost 50% of the patients who receive it.

Myeloma and related diseases (including B cell lymphoproliferative disorders) cause a variety of clinically significant hemostatic abnormalities (6). Hyperviscosity from IgM > IgA > IgG (a blood viscosity of more than 5 centipoise is a reasonable indication for plasmapheresis) leads to both arterial and venous thrombosis, particularly in the cerebral and pulmonary circulation. The paraprotein itself can affect platelet function and fibrin polymerization and inhibit the activity of endogenous von Willebrand factor. When amyloidosis develops, there can be severe factor X and sometimes factor IX depletion due to these factors binding to amyloid fibrils, and these deficiencies are relatively refractory to replacement therapy. All of the conditions described above are treated with cytotoxic chemotherapy directed at reducing the burden of malignant plasma cells.

Leukemia patients suffer life-threatening hemorrhages that in some series account for greater than 40% of acute leukemia–related deaths. In most cases bleeding is related to several factors, the most important of which is thrombocytopenia (see Chapter 14). Both acute nonlymphocytic leukemia and acute lymphocytic leukemia are associated with DIC, related to the procoagulant properties of leukemia cells. DIC can be associated in up to 10% to 20% of leukemias except acute promyelocytic leukemia (APL), where DIC is observed in almost 100% of patients.

DIC associated with APL is potentially very dangerous. To reduce this danger, the standard treatment for APL now includes the use of all-trans-retinoic acid (ATRA) before conventional induction chemotherapy. ATRA induces the differentiation of the promyelocytes into neutrophils, and this process eliminates the procoagulant and fibrinolytic properties of the leukemic cells (7). By eliminating the coagulopathic nature of the APL blasts, ATRA greatly reduces the risk of severe DIC and improves survival in this type of leukemia.

The Patient with Liver Disease

The liver is the site of production of all coagulation proteins except von Willebrand factor. It is also where ATIII, protein C, and protein S are synthesized. It clears fibrin-split products (FSPs) and D-dimers from the blood. Its blood flow is in series with the spleen, and elevated portal vein pressures are transmitted back to the spleen, which becomes engorged and sequesters blood cells, including platelets. The result is that liver disease is associated with **deficiencies of all coagulation factors**, disordered post-translational modification affecting carboxylation (of factors II, VII, IX, and X) and carbohydration (of fibrinogen leading to **dysfibrinogenemia**), **acquired ATIII deficiency, circulating anticoagulants** (FSPs and D-dimers), **a DIC-like picture, thrombocytopenia**, and a **qualitative platelet abnormality**. Defective carboxylation and dysfibrinogenemia occur with any form of liver injury and can be seen early in the course of chronic liver disease. Deficiencies of all of the coagulation factors and thrombocytopenia tend to reflect more advanced cirrhotic disease. A DIC-like picture usually means that the cirrhosis is advanced or that there is more acute injury on top of chronic cirrhosis. Bleeding often accompanies advanced liver disease.

The diagnosis of the coagulopathy of liver disease is based on the overall clinical picture. An elevated PT, aPTT, and/or thrombin time that corrects with mixing develops. In this setting, liver disease is distinguishable from vitamin K deficiency by measuring factors V and VII: both are decreased in liver disease but only FVII is decreased by vitamin K deficiency. In more advanced settings, fibrinogen falls, circulating D-dimers emerge, and thrombocytopenia worsens. At this point, liver disease is distinguishable from DIC by the bedside examination: a patient with severe liver disease who has no other reason to have DIC does not have DIC. In addition, liver disease doesn't usually cause a microangiopathic hemolytic anemia.

The treatment of the coagulopathy of liver disease is supportive. Vitamin K does not work, but plasma, cryoprecipitate, and platelets can be used judiciously in bleeding patients who require them. The nonspecific hemostatic agent desmopressin sometimes works, but one must be careful about water retention. ε-Aminocaproic acid is contraindicated in persons with advanced liver disease because it can turn a chemical DIC into clinically significant DIC.

The Uremic Patient

Bleeding in uremia is mainly due to a **qualitative platelet abnormality**. Dialysis and maintaining a hematocrit of 9 to 10 usually render this problem insignificant. If an invasive procedure is planned or if bleeding develops despite these measures, desmopressin is the treatment-of-choice (see Chapter 15).

The Patient with Disseminated Intravascular Coagulation

DIC is always a secondary event and the treatment of DIC occurs passively with the treatment of the underlying condition (8). DIC occurs secondary to severe trauma. It is particularly commonly associated with brain injury (which exposes the blood to the rich fields of lipids and tissue factor present in the brain) and large bone fractures associated with fat embolism (which triggers a systemic inflammatory response that results in the induction of expression of tissue factor on healthy endothelial cells and monocytes). DIC is also associated with sepsis, cancer, and obstetric emergencies. DIC can complicate snake and spider bites, and it develops in severe systemic inflammatory states such as anaphylaxis, transfusion reaction, and complicated bone marrow and solid organ transplants.

DIC leads to hyperactive thrombin generation and the consumption of coagulation proteins. The mechanism by which this is triggered depends on the etiology of the DIC. In general, however, thrombosis occurs because there is also the consumption of the natural anticoagulants (ATIII, protein C, and tissue factor pathway inhibitor), which seem to be relatively more depleted (or dysfunctional) than are the procoagulant factors.

In the early stage, elevated levels of plasminogen activator inhibitor-1 (PAI-1) are observed, probably as a consequence of a generalized state of cytokine "storm," which inhibits fibrinolysis and further promotes the prothrombotic response. The intravascular thrombosis also consumes platelets, resulting in thrombocytopenia, and damages red cells, resulting in a microangiopathic hemolytic anemia with circulating schistocytes. These pathophysiologic changes are reflected in the laboratory workup: elevated PT and aPTT that do not correct with mixing, thrombocytopenia that does not correct with transfusion, and anemia associated with distinctive changes in red cell morphology on blood smear. Fibrinogen levels may or may not be low because fibrinogen is an acute phase reactant and its production often counterbalances its consumption. Similarly, FSPs or D-dimers are not always elevated, depending on the amount of released PAI-1 and the PAI-1 reserve.

The treatment of DIC is geared toward the clinical manifestations of the process: one treats the complications of DIC when they arise but otherwise treatment targets the underlying problem. A bleeding patient should have platelets, coagulation factors, and fibrinogen repleted as needed. In a patient who is suffering thromboses, heparin should be administered at a low dose of 300 to 500 U/hour without a loading bolus. A patient receiving heparin should have the level of ATIII measured and repleted if it is low. ATIII may in fact be generally useful in some types of DIC, as there are data suggesting that pharmacologic doses of ATIII improve survival in septic patients (8). DIC-associated thrombosis may be the only clinical condition managed by the simultaneous administration of heparin and fresh frozen plasma: when a patient is both bleeding and clotting, hemostasis should be restored by blood product support to minimize heparin-associated bleeding.

Annotated Bibliography

1. Kearon C, Hirsh J. Management of anticoagulation before and after elective surgery. New Eng J Med 1997;336:1506–1511.

   An excellent review of the theory and practice of operating on patients who require antithrombotic therapy.

2. Brill Edwards P, Ginsberg JS, Gent M, et al. Safety of withholding heparin in pregnant women with a history of venous thromboembolism. New Engl J Med 2000;343:1439–1444.

   This study examined 125 pregnant women with a single previous episode of VTE. Antepartum heparin was withheld. Anticoagulation with subcutaneous unfractionated heparin started within 72 hours of delivery and warfarin targeting an INR of 2.0–3.0 was continued for 4 to 6 weeks. Three of the 125 women had an antepartum recurrence of VTE. The recurrences only affected women whose exhibited laboratory evidence of either thrombophilia or a previous episode of idiopathic VTE (3 of 51).

3. Brenner B. Inherited thrombophilia and pregnancy loss. Thromb Haemost 1999;82:634–640.

   An important emerging subject is presented in review format, including the investigator's experience managing women with recurrent fetal loss who were subsequently diagnosed with an inherited thrombophilia.

4. Kelton JG, Neame PB, Gauldie J, Hirsh J. Elevated platelet-associated IgG in the thrombocytopenia of septicemia. New Eng J Med 1979;300:760–764.

   Thrombocytopenia frequently accompanies bacteremia without DIC. In this study, 21 of 46 patients with bacteremia had low platelet counts, including platelets below 30,000/μL. Thrombocytopenia occurred with equal frequency with gram-negative and gram-positive organisms. Thrombocytopenia was associated with elevated platelet IgG.

5. Hutten B, Prins MH, Gent M, et al. Incidence of recurrent thromboembolism and bleeding complications among patients with venous thromboembolism in relation to both malignancy and achieved INR: a retrospective analysis. J Clin Oncol 2000;18:3078–3083.

   This retrospective analysis looked at 264 patients with cancer. The recurrence risk was 27 per 100 patients per year, and the bleeding risk was 13 per 100 patients per year. A therapeutic INR did not appear to influence the recurrence rate.

6. Glaspy JA. Hemostatic abnormalities in multiple myeloma and related disorders. In: Bick RL, ed. Hematology-Oncology Clinics of North America:

Perplexing thrombotic and hemorrhagic disorders. Philadelphia: Saunders, 1992:1301–1314.

An encyclopedic review of the subject.

7. Menell JS, Cesarman GM, Jacovina AT, et al. Annexin II and bleeding in acute promyelocytic leukemia (APL). New Engl J Med 1999;340:994–1004.

Annexin II on APL cells binds to tissue plasminogen activator and plasminogen. An APL cell is therefore a tiny carrier of fibrinolytic activity. All-trans-retinoic acid (ATRA) eliminated the surface expression of annexin II and cell-associated fibrinolytic activity. This may be a reason why ATRA treats APL-associated DIC.

8. Levi M, Ten Cate H. Disseminated intravascular coagulation. New Engl J Med 1999;341:586–592.

A recent review of a subject that everyone knows a little about but needs to learn more about.

Index

Note: Pages numbers with an *f* indicate figures; those with a *t* indicate tables.